SOAP
for
Family Medicine

Look for other books in this series!

SOAP
for
Family Medicine

Daniel C. Maldonado, MD

Assistant Clinical Professor
Department of Family Medicine
University of Southern California, Keck School of Medicine
Los Angeles, California
Attendng Physician of Family Medicine
Assistant Director of Inpatient Medicine
White Memorial Medical Center (WMMC)
WMMC Family Practice Residency Program
Los Angeles, California

Cynthia Zúñiga, MD

Assistant Clinical Professor
Department of Family Medicine
University of Southern California, Keck School of Medicine
Los Angeles, California
Attending Physician of Family Medicine
White Memorial Medical Center (WMMC)
WMMC Family Practice Residency Program
Los Angeles, California

Series Editor:
Peter S. Uzelac, MD, FACOG

Assistant Professor
Department of Obstetrics and Gynecology
University of Southern California, Keck School of Medicine
Los Angeles, California

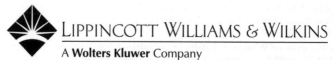

LIPPINCOTT WILLIAMS & WILKINS
A **Wolters Kluwer** Company
Philadelphia • Baltimore • New York • London
Buenos Aires • Hong Kong • Sydney • Tokyo

351 West Camden Street
Baltimore, Maryland 21201-2436 USA

530 Walnut Street
Philadelphia, Pennsylvania 19106-3621 USA

ISBN-13: 978-1-4051-0437-1
ISBN-10: 1-4051-0437-6

Library of Congress Cataloging-in-Publication Data

Maldonado, Daniel C., M.D.
    SOAP for family medicine / Daniel C. Maldonado, Cynthis Zúñiga. – 1st ed.
        p. ; cm.
    Includes index.
    ISBN 1-4051-0437-6 (pbk.)
    1. Medical protocols–Handbooks, manuals, etc.   2. Family medicine–
Handbooks, manuals, etc.
    [DNLM: 1. Family Pactice–Handbooks. WB 39 M244s 2005]
    I. Zúñiga, Cynthia.   II. Title.
    RC64.M25   2005
    610–dc22
                                                        2004013260

A catalogue record for this title is available from the British Library

Editor: Donna Balado
Managing Editor: Kathleen Scogna
Marketing Manager: Emilie Linkins

To purchase additional copies of this book call our customer service department at (800) 638-3030 or fax orders to (301) 824-7390. International customers should call (301) 714-2324.

Visit **Lippincott Williams & Wilkins on the Internet: http://www.lww.com.** Lippincott Williams & Wilkins customer service representatives are available from 8:30 am to 6:00 pm, EST, Monday through Friday, for telephone access.

17

In memory of my brother, James, whose spirit is with us every day. To my parents for all the love and support they have given me over the years. To all my siblings, who have inspired me in one way or another.

DCM

To my loving parents, Amelia and Enrique, who have taught me the valuable lessons of life. To all my teachers, who have inspired me to learn. To all my patients, who continue making medicine a challenge.

CZ

Contents

To the Reader

Like most medical students, I started my ward experience head down and running, eager to finally make contact with real patients. What I found was a confusing world, completely different from anything I had known during the first two years of medical school. New language, foreign abbreviations, and residents too busy to set my bearings straight: Where would I begin?

Pocket textbooks, offering medical knowledge in a convenient and portable package, seemed to be the logical solution. Unfortunately, I found myself spending valuable time sifting through large amounts of text, often not finding the answer to my question, and in the process missing out on teaching points during rounds!

I designed the SOAP series to provide medical students and house staff with pocket manuals that truly serve their intended purpose: quick accessibility to the most practical clinical information in a user-friendly format. At the inception of this project, I envisioned all of the benefits the SOAP format would bring to the reader:

- Learning through this model reinforces a thought process that is already familiar to students and residents, facilitating easier long-term retention.

- SOAP promotes good communication between physicians and facilitates the teaching/learning process.

- SOAP puts the emphasis back on the patient's clinical problem and not the diagnosis.

- In the age of managed care, SOAP meets the challenge of providing efficiency while maintaining quality.

- As sound medical-legal practice gains attention in physician training, SOAP emphasizes adherence to a documentation style that leaves little room for potential misinterpretation.

Rather than attempting to summarize the contents of a thousand-page textbook into a miniature form, the SOAP series focuses exclusively on guidance through patient encounters. In a typical use, "finding out where to start" or "refreshing your memory" with SOAP books should be possible in less than a minute. Subjects are always confined to two pages, and the most important points have been highlighted. Topics have been limited to those problems you will most commonly encounter repeatedly during your training, and contents are grouped according to the hospital or clinic setting. Facts and figures that are not particularly helpful to surviving life on the wards, such as demographics, pathophysiology, and busy tables and graphs have purposely been omitted (such details are much better studied in a quiet environment using large and comprehensive texts).

Congratulations on your achievements thus far, and I wish you a highly successful medical career!

Peter S. Uzelac, MD, FACOG

Acknowledgments

We would like to thank White Memorial Medical Center's Family Practice Residency Program and Family Care Specialists Medical Group for their continued commitment to training family practice physicians in the underserved population. Additionally, we would like to thank Peter Uzelac for providing us with the opportunity and guidance to write this manual. Special thanks to Blackwell Publishing and their staff (especially Selene Steneck) for their tremendous support and patience throughout this project.

Reviewers

Catarina Castañeda
Class of 2004
Drexel University College of Medicine
Philadelphia, Pennsylvania

Richard Ian Gray
Class of 2005
University of Tennessee Health Science Center College of Medicine
Memphis, Tennessee

Susan Merel
Class of 2005
University of Chicago Pritzker School of Medicine
Chicago, Illinois

Ngoc Phan
Class of 2004
Harvard University School of Medicine
Boston, Massachusetts

Rebecca Smith
Class of 2005
University of California, Irvine College of Medicine
Irvine, California

Abbreviations

ABC	airway, breathing, circulation
ABG	arterial blood gas
AC	acromioclavicular
ACE	angiotensin-converting enzymes
ACL	anterior cruciate ligament
AD	atopic dermatitis
ADA	American Diabetes Association
ADHD	attention-deficit/hyperactivity disorder
AGE	acute gastroenteritis
AK	actinic keratosis
ANA	antinuclear antibody
AR	allergic rhinitis
ARB	angiotensin-II receptor blockers
ASD	atrial septal defect
BCC	basal cell carcinoma
bid	*bis in die* (twice daily)
β-hCG	beta human chorionic gonadotropin
BMI	body mass index
BP	blood pressure
BPH	benign prostatic hyperplasia
BUN	blood urea nitrogen
CAD	coronary artery disease
CBC	complete blood count
CDC	Centers for Disease Control and Prevention
CHD	coronary heart disease
COPD	chronic obstructive pulmonary disease
COX	cyclooxygenase
CPR	cardiopulmonary resuscitation
CRP	C-reactive protein
CSF	cerebral spinal fluid
CT	computed tomography
CVAT	costovertebral angle tenderness
CXR	chest x-ray
DASH	dietary approaches to stop hypertension
DIP	distal interphalangeal
DSM-IV	Diagnostic and Statistical Manual of Mental Disorders
DUB	dysfunctional uterine bleeding
EBV	Epstein-Barr virus
ECG	electrocardiogram
ENT	ears, nose, throat
ER	emergency room
ESR	erythrocyte sedimentation rate
FEV_1	forced expiratory volume at 1 second
FMH	family medical history
FSH	follicle-stimulating hormone
FOBT	fecal occult blood test
GBS	group B streptococcus

GERD	gastroesophageal reflux disease
GH	glenohumeral
GHM	general health maintenance
GI	gastrointestinal
GIB	gastrointestinal bleed
HDL	high-density lipoprotein
HEADSSS	home, education, activities, drugs, sexuality, safety, suicide
HEENT	head, ears, eyes, nose, throat
HIDA	dimethyl iminodiacetic acid
HIV	human immunodeficiency virus
HPI	history of present illness
HPV	human papilloma virus
HR	heart rate
HRT	hormone replacement therapy
HSV	herpes simplex virus
IM	intramuscular
IUD	intrauterine device
IV	intravenous
JNC	Joint National Committee
JVD	jugular venous distention
KOH	potassium hydroxide
KUB	kidney, ureter, bladder
LD	Lyme disease
LDH	lactate dehydrogenase
LDL	low-density lipoprotein
LFTs	liver function tests
LH	luteinizing hormone
LRI	lower respiratory infection
MMR	measles/mumps/rubella
MRI	magnetic resonance imaging
NPH	isophane insulin
NPO	*nulla per os* (nothing by mouth)
NSAIDs	nonsteroidal anti-inflammatory drugs
OA	osteoarthritis
Ob/Gyn	obstetric/gynecology
PA/LAT	posterior-anterior/lateral
PCOS	polycystic ovarian syndrome
PDA	patent ductus arteriosus
PEF	peak expiratory flow
PGF	prostaglandin F
PID	pelvic inflammatory disease
PIP	proximal interphalangeal
PMDD	premenstrual dysphoric disorder
PMH	past medical history
PMI	point of maximum impulse
PMS	premenstrual syndrome
PO	*per os* (by mouth)
PPD	purified protein derivative
PSA	prostate specific antigen
PSH	past surgical history

pt	patient
PT	prothrombin time
PTT	partial thromboplastin time
PUD	peptic ulcer disease
PUVA	psoralen ultraviolet A
qd	*quaque die* (once daily)
qid	*quater in die* (four times daily)
RBC	red blood cell
RF	rheumatoid factor
RLQ	right lower quadrant
ROS	review of systems
RPR	rapid plasma reagin
RR	respiratory rate
RSV	respiratory syncytial virus
RUDS	random urine drug screen
RUQ	right upper quadrant
SCC	squamous cell carcinoma
SH	social history
SIDS	sudden infant death syndrome
SPAK	spreading pigmented actinic keratosis
SSRI	selective serotonin reuptake inhibitor
STD	sexually transmitted disease
STI	sexually transmitted infection
TB	tuberculosis
TIA	transient ischemic attack
tid	*ter in die* (thrice daily)
TIPS	transjugular intrahepatic portosystemic shunt
TMJ	temporomandibular joint
TSH	thyroid-stimulating hormone
TSI	thyroid-stimulating immunoglobulin
UA	urinalysis
URI	upper respiratory infection
UTI	urinary tract infection
UV	ultraviolet
UVA	ultraviolet A
UVB	ultraviolet B
VCUG	voiding cystourethrogram
VDRL	venereal disease research laboratory
VSD	ventricular septal defect
WBC	white blood cell

Normal Lab Values

Blood, Plasma, Serum

Aminotransferase, alanine (ALT, SGPT)	0–35 U/L
Aminotransferase, aspartate (AST, SGOT)	0–35 U/L
Ammonia, plasma	40–80 µg/dL
Amylase, serum	0–130 U/L
Antistreptolysin O titer	Less than 150 units
Bicarbonate, serum	23–28 meq/L
Bilirubin, serum	
Total	0.3–1.2 mg/dL
Direct	0–0.3 mg/dL
Blood gases, arterial (room air)	
PO_2	80–100 mm Hg
PCO_2	35–45 mm Hg
pH	7.38–7.44
Calcium, serum	9.0–10.5 mg/dL
Carbon dioxide content, serum	23–28 meq/L
Chloride, serum	98–106 meq/L
Cholesterol, total, plasma	150–199 mg/dL (desirable)
Cholesterol, low-density lipoprotein (LDL), plasma	$\leq$ 130 mg/dL (desirable)
Cholesterol, high-density lipoprotein (HDL), plasma	$\geq$ 40 mg/dL (desirable)
Complement, serum	
C3	55–120 mg/dL
Total	37–55 U/mL
Copper, serum	70–155 µg/dL
Creatine kinase, serum	30–170 U/L
Creatinine, serum	0.7–1.3 mg/dL
Ethanol, blood	< 50 mg/dL
Fibrinogen, plasma	150–350 mg/dL
Folate, red cell	160–855 ng/mL
Folate, serum	2.5–20 ng/mL
Glucose, plasma	
Fasting	70–105 mg/dL
2 hours postprandial	< 140 mg/dL
Iron, serum	60–160 µg/dL
Iron-binding capacity, serum	250–460 µg/dL
Lactate dehydrogenase, serum	60–100 U/L
Lactic acid, venous blood	6–16 mg/dL
Lead, blood	< 40 µg/dL

Lipase, serum	< 95 U/L
Magnesium, serum	1.5–2.4 mg/dL
Manganese, serum	0.3–0.9 ng/mL
Methylmalonic acid, serum	150–370 nmol/L
Osmolality plasma	275–295 mosm/kg H_2O
Phosphatase, acid, serum	0.5–5.5 U/L
Phosphatase, alkaline, serum	36–92 U/L
Phosphorus, inorganic, serum	3.0–4.5 mg/dL
Potassium, serum	3.5–5.0 meq/L
Protein, serum	
Total	6.0–7.8 g/dL
Albumin	3.5–5.5 g/dL
Globulins	2.5–3.5 g/dL
$Alpha_1$	0.2–0.4 g/dL
$Alpha_2$	0.5–0.9 g/dL
Beta	0.6–1.1 g/dL
Gamma	0.7–1.7 g/dL
Rheumatoid factor	< 40 U/mL
Sodium, serum	136–145 meq/L
Triglycerides	< 150 mg/dL (desirable)
Urea nitrogen, serum	8–20 mg/dL
Uric acid, serum	2.5–8 mg/dL
Vitamin B_{12}, serum	200–800 pg/mL

Cerebrospinal Fluid

Cell count	0–5 cells/μL
Glucose (less than 40% of simultaneous plasma concentration is abnormal)	40–80 mg/dL
Protein	15–60 mg/dL
Pressure (opening)	70–200 cm H_2O

Endocrine

Adrenocorticotropin (ACTH)	9–52 pg/mL
Aldosterone, serum	
Supine	2–5 ng/dL
Standing	7–20 ng/dL
Aldosterone, urine	5–19 μg/24 hours
Cortisol	
Serum 8 AM	8–20 μg/dL
5 PM	3–13 μg/dL

1 hour after cosyntropin usually ≥ 8 µg/dL above baseline	> 18 µg/dL
Overnight suppression test	< 5 µg/dL
Urine free cortisol	< 90 µg/24 hours
Estradiol, serum	
Male	10–30 pg/mL
Female	
Cycle day 1–10	50–100 pmol/L
Cycle day 11–20	50–200 pmol/L
Cycle day 21–30	70–150 pmol/L
Estriol, urine	> 12 mg/24 hours
Follicle-stimulating hormone, serum	
Male (adult)	5–15 mU/mL
Female	
Follicular or luteal phase	5–20 mU/mL
Midcycle peak	30–50 mU/mL
Postmenopausal	> 35 mU/mL
Insulin, serum (fasting)	5–20 mU/L
17-ketosteroids, urine	
Male	8–22 mg/24 hours
Female	Up to 15 µg/24 hours
Luteinizing hormone, serum	
Male	3–15 mU/mL (3–15 U/L)
Female	
Follicular or luteal phase	5–22 mU/mL
Midcycle peak	30–250 mU/mL
Postmenopausal	> 30 mU/mL
Parathyroid hormone, serum	10–65 pg/mL
Progesterone	
Luteal	3–30 ng/mL
Follicular	< 1 ng/mL
Prolactin, serum	
Male	< 15 ng/mL
Female	< 20 ng/mL
Testosterone, serum	
Adult male	300–1200 ng/dL
Female	20–75 ng/dL
Thyroid function tests (normal ranges vary)	
Thyroid iodine (^{131}I) uptake	10%–30% of administered dose at 24 hours

Thyroid-stimulating hormone (TSH)	0.5–5.0 μU/mL
Thyroxine (T4), serum	
Total	5–12 pg/dL
Free	0.9–2.4 ng/dL
Free T4 index	4–11
Triiodothyronine, resin (T3)	25%–35%
Triiodothyronine, serum (T3)	70–195 ng/dL
Vitamin D	
1,25-dihydroxy, serum	25–65 pg/mL
25-hydroxy, serum	15–80 ng/mL

Gastrointestinal

Fecal urobilinogen	40–280 mg/24 hours
Gastrin, serum	0–180 pg/mL
Lactose tolerance test	
Increase in plasma glucose	> 15 mg/dL
Lipase, ascitic fluid	< 200 U/L
Secretin-cholecystokinin pancreatic function	> 80 meq/L of HCO_3 in at least 1 specimen collected over 1 hour
Stool fat	< 5 g/d on a 100-g fat diet
Stool nitrogen	< 2 g/d
Stool weight	< 200 g/d

Hematology

Activated partial thromboplastin time	25–35 seconds
Bleeding time	< 10 minutes
Coagulation factors, plasma	
Factor I	150–350 mg/dL
Factor II	60%–150% of normal
Factor V	60%–150% of normal
Factor VII	60%–150% of normal
Factor VIII	60%–150% of normal
Factor IX	60%–150% of normal
Factor X	60%–150% of normal
Factor XI	60%–150% of normal
Factor XII	60%–150% of normal
Erythrocyte count	4.2–5.9 million cells/μL
Erythropoietin	< 30 mU/mL
D-dimer	< 0.5 μg/mL

Ferritin, serum	15–200 ng/mL
Glucose-6-phosphate dehydrogenase, blood	5–15 U/g Hgb
Haptoglobin, serum	50–150 mg/dL
Hematocrit	
Male	41%–51%
Female	36%–47%
Hemoglobin, blood	
Male	14–17 g/dL
Female	12–16 g/dL
Hemoglobin, plasma	0.5–5 mg/dL
Leukocyte alkaline phosphatase	15–40 mg of phosphorus liberated/ hour per 10^{10} cells
Score	13–130/100 polymorphonuclear neutrophils and band forms
Leukocyte count	
Nonblacks	4000–10,000/μL
Blacks	3500–10,000/μL
Lymphocytes	
CD4+ cell count	640–1175/μL
CD8+ cell count	335–875/μL
CD4 : CD8 ratio	1.0–4.0
Mean corpuscular hemoglobin (MCH)	28–32 pg
Mean corpuscular hemoglobin concentration (MCHC)	32–36 g/dL
Mean corpuscular volume (MCV)	80–100 fL
Platelet count	150,000–350,000/μL
Protein C activity, plasma	67%–131%
Protein C resistance	2.2–2.6
Protein S activity, plasma	82%–144%
Prothrombin time	11–13 s
Reticulocyte count	0.5%–1.5% of erythrocytes
Absolute	23,000–90,000 cells/μL
Schilling test (oral administration of radioactive cobalamin-labeled vitamin B_{12})	8.5%–28% excreted in urine per 24–48 h
Sedimentation rate, erythrocyte (Westergren)	
Male	0–15 mm/hour
Female	0–20 mm/hour

Volume, blood
  Plasma
    Male   25–44 mL/kg body weight
    Female   28–43 mL/kg body weight
  Erythrocyte
    Male   25–35 mL/kg body weight
    Female   20–30 mL/kg body weight

Urine

Amino acids	200–400 mg/24 hours
Amylase	6.5–48.1 U/hour
Calcium	100–300 mg/d on unrestricted diet
Chloride	80–250 meq/d (varies with intake)
Copper	0–100 μg/24 hours
Creatine	
Male	4–40 mg/24 hours
Female	0–100 mg/24 hours
Creatinine	15–25 mg/kg per 24 hours
Creatinine clearance	90–140 mL/min
Osmolality	38–1400 mosm/kg H_2O
Phosphate, tubular resorption	79%–94% (0.79–0.94) of filtered load
Potassium	25–100 meq/24 hours (varies with intake)
Protein	< 100 mg/24 hours
Sodium	100–260 meq/24 hours (varies with intake)
Uric acid	250–750 mg/24 hours (varies with diet)
Urobilinogen	0.05–2.5 mg/24 hours

I

Medicine

S Obtain identifying data
Pt age, gender, and marital status

Obtain a full history
HPI: Obtain a complete history of the pt's illness.
- Refer to specific topics for guidance.

PMH: List any medical problems, including adult and childhood illnesses, and hospitalizations.

FMH: Obtain the health status and age of relatives.
- Living or deceased relatives with medical conditions

PSH: Has the pt had any surgeries or minor procedures?

SH:
- Ask about tobacco, alcohol, or drug use.
- Obtain an exercise and diet history.
- What is the pt's occupation? What is the pt's education level?
- Review daily life activities; home situation; level of functioning.
- List activities or hobbies.
- Document pt's beliefs or religion.
- Review pt safety measures (e.g., smoke detectors, seat belts, and helmets).
- Obtain a sexual history:
  - Having sex with men, women, or both?
  - How many lifetime partners?
  - Any history of sexually transmitted diseases?

Ob/Gyn: Collect pregnancy, menstruation, pap smear, breast exam, mammogram, and contraception histories.

Medications: List current medications, supplements, vitamins, and herbal supplements.

Allergies: Is the pt allergic to any medications, foods, or other substances?
- What is the reaction with each allergy?

Immunizations: Review pt's immunization status.

Perform ROS
General: Any weight loss or gain, weakness, fatigue, or fever?

HEENT:
- Ask about headaches, syncope, or dizziness.
- Does the pt use corrective lenses or have visual changes?
- Document hearing problems.
- Nose or sinus conditions?
- Any problems with the teeth, tongue, or throat?
- Lymphadenopathy or neck masses?

Breast: Does the pt have complaints of lumps, pain, or discharge?

Respiratory: Any shortness of breath, dyspnea on exertion, wheezing, or cough?

Cardiac: Any complaint of chest pain, palpitations, orthopnea, edema, paroxysmal nocturnal dyspnea, or other heart problems?

Gastrointestinal:
- Has the pt experienced abdominal pain, melena, rectal bleeding, or hemoptysis?
- Any nausea, dysphagia, vomiting, diarrhea, or constipation?
- Does the pt have liver-related symptoms such as jaundice, icterus, or bleeding?

Urinary: Complaint of dysuria, frequency, urgency, nocturia, hematuria, or incontinence?

Genital: Does the pt complain of genital symptoms?

Musculoskeletal: Joint/muscle pain, weakness, injuries, or conditions?
Neurologic: Has there been numbness, seizures, blackouts, or paralysis?
Hematologic: History of anemia, bleeding, bruising, or blood transfusion?
Endocrine: Any hypo-/hyperthyroid or hypo-/hypergylcemia symptoms?
Skin: Are there complaints of rashes, lesions, or nail changes?
Psychiatric:
  • Review psychiatric history for depression, anxiety, suicide ideation, or plan.
  • Auditory or visual hallucinations in the past or present?

O **Check vital signs**
Height, weight, body mass index
Blood pressure should be checked yearly.

Perform physical exam
Full physical to include clinical breast exam, rectal, and pelvic exam when indicated
See specific topics for detailed exam instructions.

Consider the following labs and studies:

- CBC	- Chemistry panel
- TSH	- Liver panel
- PSA	- RPR
- Fecal occult blood test (FOBT)	- CXR
- ECG	- Papanicolaou test
- Lipid panel	

A **Adult History & Physical, Preventive Maintenance**

P **Employ preventive measures**
Screen for breast cancer
  • Breast self-exam: Monthly
  • Mammogram: Starting at age 40 every 1 to 2 years
Screen for colorectal cancer
  • FOBT: Starting at age 50 annually
  • Flexible sigmoidoscopy: Starting at age 50 every 5 years
  • Colonoscopy: Starting age 50 every 10 years
    ◆ If there is a 1st-degree relative with colorectal cancer, start at age 40
Screen for cervical cancer
  • Papanicolaou test: Every one to three years depending on risk
    ◆ May need to be done more frequently if abnormality detected
    ◆ Begin at the age when pt becomes sexually active or at age 21 (whichever comes first)
    ◆ Can discontinue at age 65 if tests have been consistently normal in the previous 10 years
Screen for testicular cancer
  • Testicular self-exam: Monthly
Screen for osteoporosis
  • Bone mineral density measurement
    ◆ Starting at age 65
    ◆ Younger if pt has risk factors
      • Previous spinal fracture, family history, low body weight, or smoker

Immunize pt
- Tetanus vaccine every 10 years
- Influenza yearly after age 50 or younger if high risk
- Pneumococcal vaccine given at age 65 or younger if high risk

Screen for hypercholesterolemia
- Check every 5 years if normal

Implement behavioral and dietary modifications
Calcium supplementation
Folic acid if pt is of childbearing age and able to become pregnant
Diet and exercise
Smoking cessation
Skin protection

Implement general health maintenance issues
Dental care: Yearly exam and cleaning
Vision care: Every 2 years at age 40 or younger if visual problems present
- Tonometry test every 2 years with exam after age 45

Hearing care: Yearly exams after age 65
Family planning if pt is of childbearing age

Preventive Maintenance Recommended by the United States Preventive Services Task Force (USPSTF) for Adults*

	|18	25	30	35	40	45	50	55	60	65	70	75
Screening												
Blood Pressure, Height & Weight	Periodically											
Obesity	Periodically											
Cholesterol				Every 5 years (Women Start at Age 45)								
Pap Smear	Women: Every 1 to 3 years											
Chlamydia	Routinely											
Mammography					Every 1 to 2 Years							
Colorectal Cancer							Depends on Test					
Alcohol Use	Periodically											
Vision & Hearing											Periodically	
Immunization												
Tetanus-Diptheria (Td)	Every 10 years											
Varicella (VZV)	Susceptibles-Two doses											
Measles, Mumps, Rubella (MMR)	Women of Childbearing Age											
Pneumococcal										One Dose		
Influenza							Yearly					
Chemoprevention												
Assess CHD risks & Aspirin Prevention				Men Periodically (Women start at Age 50)								
Counseling												
Calcium Intake	Women: Periodically											
Folic Acid/Breastfeeding	Women of Childbearing Age/Women After Childbirth											
Tobacco, drug, alcohol, STIs, HIV, Exercise, Sun Exposure, Oral Health, Safety, Medications	Periodically											

*Recommendation from USPSTF at www.preventiveservices.ahrq.gov

S **What are the pt's complaints?**
Allergic rhinitis (AR) can present with clear rhinorrhea, paroxysms of sneezing, and pruritus of the palate or nose.
If no pruritus or paroxysms of sneezing, consider eosinophilic or vasomotor rhinitis.
Consider sinusitis if there are symptoms of headache, halitosis, and purulent nasal discharge.

Review the timing of the symptoms
Perennial or yearlong allergies are usually related to indoor allergens.
Seasonal allergies are usually related to pollen or aeroallergens in the air.

Can the pt breathe through both nares?
If pt has difficulty breathing through either or both nares, consider obstruction, polyps, septal deviation, or inflammation of the turbinates.

Are there any environmental factors triggering AR?
Common triggers include pets, aeroallergens, occupational pollutants or chemicals, indoor dust/mites/cockroaches, first- or second-hand smoke, foods, meds, etc.
Weekly household vacuuming, dusting, and changing or washing of bedding are important in reducing symptoms of AR.

How much fluid intake is the pt receiving each day?
Proper hydration reduces symptoms.

O **Perform physical exam**
General: Mouth breathing suggests nasal airway obstruction.
HEENT:
- Nasal mucosa can be pale to gray-bluish, boggy, and with clear discharge.
- Nonallergic or vasomotor rhinitis may have red mucosa.
- Check for injected sclera, which may indicate allergic conjunctivitis.
- *Dark circles under the eyes are called "allergic shiners."*
- *"Cobblestoning" of the oropharyngeal mucosa is caused by inflammation from chronic postnasal drip.*
- *A horizontal nasal crease is caused by repetitive upward nasal manipulation, also known as the "nasal salute."*

Chest: Auscultate chest for presence of wheezing because many pts with asthma have allergies.
Skin: Check for any rashes or hives.

Consider the following labs or studies if severe AR:
Skin testing if a specific allergen is suspected
Nasal smear for eosinophils can be diagnostic for eosinophilic AR
Serum IgE radioallergosorbent test if severe dermatographism or eczema present

Allergic Rhinitis
Types: Seasonal and perennial allergic rhinitis

Differential Diagnosis
Vasomotor (nonallergic) rhinitis
Medicamentosa rhinitis (Usually there is a history of chronic decongestant use.)

Implement environmental controls to minimize or remove allergens
Minimize indoor exposures with dustproof covers on mattresses and pillows.
- Dust furniture with a damp towel.
- Wash floors with a damp mop.
- Remove or minimize carpeting.
- Keep home humidified less than 50%.
- Remove pets from home if allergic.
- Wash bedding once a week in hot water.

Minimize outdoor allergies by having pt avoid any gardening.
- Home windows should be closed.
- Air conditioning can be used.
- Avoid activities that may expose pt to aeroallergens.

Prescribe medication
Antihistamines can be used to reduce sneezing, itching, or rhinorrhea.
- First generation antihistamines cause sedation and are available over-the-counter.
- Second generation antihistamines have less sedation:
    - Loratadine (Claritin)   - Cetrizine (Zyrtec)
    - Fexofenadine (Allegra)   - Desloratadine (Clarinex)
    - Azelastine (Astelin) nasal spray
- If nasal congestion is present, a decongestant such as pseudoephedrine (Sudafed) can be added with above medicine or in combination form.

For long-term control of allergic rhinitis, use nasally inhaled corticosteroids:
    - Triamcinolone (Nasocort)   - Fluticasone (Flonase)
    - Beclomethasone (Vancenase)   - Budesonide (Rhinocort)
    - Flunisolide (Nasarel)   - Cromolyn (Nasalcrom)
Leukotriene receptor antagonists may have some benefit.
Omalizumab is a monoclonal recombinant antibody for anti-IgE therapy.

Begin trial of immunotherapy if severe AR
Referral to an allergist is recommended.
Immunotherapy is indicated for severe allergies and has been shown to reduce symptoms markedly.

Initiate hydration with up to eight 8-oz. glasses of noncaffeinated fluids per day to reduce symptoms.

S **Does the pt present with symptoms of anemia?**
Symptoms can be dizziness, fatigue, palpitations, shortness of breath, dyspnea on exertion, and pica.

Are there signs of bleeding?
GI blood loss can be seen as melena, hematochezia, hemoptysis, or rectal bleeding. Vaginal bleeding from uterine fibroids or heavy menstruation can cause anemia.

Review dietary intake of iron-fortified foods
Children can be especially vulnerable for anemia without proper nutrition.

Is there a family history of bleeding disorders?
There are many types of genetic disorders that cause anemia, such as sickle cell, hemophilia, or thalassemia.

Has there been exposure to lead?
Lead poisoning can cause basophilic stippling of the red blood cells (RBCs).

Is the pt pregnant or lactating?
There is an increased demand for iron during these states.

Does the pt have a history of gastric or small bowel surgery?
These pts may have difficulty absorbing iron.

Is there any history or evidence of hemolysis?
This can be seen in idiopathic pulmonary hemosiderosis, paroxysmal nocturnal hemoglobinuria, or in abnormal heart valves causing trauma to RBCs.

O **Check vital signs**
Check orthostatic vitals to confirm hemodynamic stability.

Perform physical exam
General: Exam is usually normal.
HEENT:
- Search for pale conjunctiva, stomatitis, cheilosis, or glossitis.
- Plummer-Vinson syndrome: dysphasia and anemia with glossitis, splenomegaly, and atrophy of the mouth, pharynx, and upper esophagus

Heart: Tachycardia or flow murmurs can be present in high-output states.
Abdomen: Splenomegaly can indicate sequestration.
Nails: Check nails for koilonychia (thin concaved nails with raised edges).
Pelvic: Perform if history of vaginal bleeding.
Rectal:
- Perform stool guaiac and digital rectal exam.
- Search for bleeding, melena, hemorrhoids, or masses.

Consider the following labs
CBC for microcytic hypochromic indices
UA for hematuria
Serum iron studies (Iron deficient = low iron level, low ferritin, and high total iron-binding capacity)
Thyroid-stimulating hormone if signs and symptoms of hypothyroidism
Peripheral smear may be indicated
Electrophoresis if thalassemia is suspected

Fecal occult blood test times three to rule out GI bleed
Lead level if any evidence of lead poisoning

 Iron-Deficiency Anemia
Possible etiologies by age:
- *Infants*: Increased iron requirements, low iron stores, microscopic blood loss, iron-deficient diets
- *Children*: Malnutrition, pica, or lead toxicity
- *Adolescents*: Rapid growth, eating disorders, and menses
- *Adults*: Gastrointestinal or urogenital bleed, menses, malnutrition or malabsorption, celiac disease, gastric or small bowel surgery, hemolysis, hypothyroidism
- *Other*: Thalassemia, anemia of chronic disease, sideroblastic anemia

 Provide iron supplementation therapy
Ferrous sulfate qd to qid for at least six months
Vitamin C can be used to help increase absorption of iron.
Increase iron-fortified foods such as red meats and leafy green vegetables.
Avoid taking with calcium, milk, and antacids because these may decrease iron absorption.
Prescribe a stool softener with iron because constipation is common.
For severe iron deficiency, hospitalization and replacement with parental iron or transfusion of packed RBCs may be required.

Refer if indicated
If GI bleed or possible malignancy, a GI referral is indicated.
- Barium enema, upper gastrointestinal series, or endoscopy may be needed.
If any evidence of hemolysis, consider hematology referral.
Pelvic bleeding may need surgical intervention from gynecology.
- Pelvic ultrasound is useful if uterine fibroids or polyps are suspected.

Implement prevention and screening
Educate pt on nutrition with iron-fortified foods along with vitamins.
Screen at-risk populations, especially children and menstruating women.

S **What are the pt's symptoms?**
The severity, quality, location, and radiation of the pain can make the diagnosis.
Usually periumbilical or midepigastric pain presents first (visceral pain).
The abdominal pain then radiates and localizes to the RLQ (parietal pain).

Are there any associated symptoms?
Commonly associated symptoms include:
- Fever   - Nausea
- Vomiting   - Anorexia
Less common symptoms may include:
- Diarrhea   - Hematemesis
- Hematochezia   - Melena
In appendicitis, pain typically presents before vomiting, the reverse being true in acute
gastroenteritis.

What makes the pain better or worse?
The pain is usually worsened with movement such as walking.
The pt may find that bending the knees toward the chest alleviates the pain.
Intermittent resolution of pain may indicate a perforated appendix.

It is unlikely that the pt has appendicitis if there is a desire to eat.

O **Check vital signs**
Low-grade temperature is commonly present.
High-grade temperature and tachycardia may indicate perforation.

Perform a physical exam
Abdomen:
- Auscultate for bowel sounds.
- Look for signs of rebound or guarding, which may indicate peritoneal
  irritation.
- *McBurney's point*: Maximum tenderness to palpation at about one-third away
  from the anterosuperior iliac spine to the umbilicus
- *Rovsing's sign*: Palpation in the LLQ elicits pain in the RLQ.
- *Obturator sign*: Pain with internal rotation of a flexed hip and knee
- *Psoas sign*: Pain with full extension of hip and knee or lifting the thigh against
  pressure
Rectal and pelvic exams should be performed.

Consider the following labs:
CBC to determine if WBCs are elevated
β-hCG to rule out pregnancy
LFTs to rule out hepatobiliary disease
UA may have mild pyuria or hematuria
Amylase, usually to determine if cause is pancreatitis; however, remember that it can be
mildly elevated with vomiting, as seen in gastroenteritis.

Consider imaging if clinical picture is vague
Abdominal radiographs: Sometimes a fecalith or sentinel loop of dilated bowel is seen
next to the appendix.
Abdominal ultrasound or spiral CT scan to visualize the appendix

Acute Appendicitis: *Remember, appendicitis is a clinical diagnosis.*
Causes:
- Fecalith usually in adults
- Lymphoid hyperplasia usually in children

Differential Diagnosis

- *Yersinia enterocolitica* infection
- Cecal diverticulitis
- Intussusception
- Mittelschmerz

- Mesenteric lymphadenitis
- Meckel's diverticulum
- Acute gastroenteritis
- Tubal ovarian cyst

P   **Admit pt to the hospital**
Keep pt NPO before surgery.
Administer IV fluids.
Start pain management.
Begin IV antibiotic therapy.

Obtain surgical consult

S

What are the frequency and severity of the pt's symptoms?
Common symptoms are wheezing, dyspnea, cough, and chest tightness.
These symptoms may be mild to severe and can occur during certain times of the day or with activities.

Determine the triggers and timing of exacerbations
Exacerbations can affect daily activities, which translate to functional days lost.
Day versus night exacerbations may give insight into a specific cause or trigger.

Has an asthma action plan been incorporated into the pt's care?
Components of an action plan include medication, response to medication, peak flow measurements, and a diary of symptoms as they relate to triggers.

Does the pt have a history of hospitalizations or ER visits?
Include any history of intubations, which may give an idea of the severity of the pt's asthma.

Does the pt have allergies?
Allergic rhinitis, dermatitis, and ectopy are all commonly associated with asthma.

Any history of recent or current illness?
Exacerbations are often caused by preceding illnesses.

O

Check vital signs
Play close attention to respiratory rate and oxygen saturation.
Severe attack = RR > 28, HR > 110 bpm and pulsus paradoxus > 12 mm Hg systolic BP drop with inspiration
Obtain peak flow measurements before and after nebulizer treatments and compare to baseline if available.

Perform physical exam
General: Severe attacks are associated with respiratory distress, difficulty speaking in full sentences, diaphoresis, and use of accessory muscles.
HEENT:
- Examine nasal mucosa and oropharyngeal mucosa for abnormalities.
- Physical findings may suggest allergic rhinitis.
Chest:
- Auscultate chest for presence of wheezing, crackles, or rales.
- Usually decreased aeration with expiratory phase > inspiratory phase.
Skin: Inspect for any rashes or hives.

Consider the following labs:
ABG usually shows respiratory alkalosis.
CXR to rule out pneumonia, pneumothorax, or atelectasis
CBC if signs of infection
Spirometry: if forced expiratory volume (FEV_1) does not improve to 40% of predicted value after treatment, the pt will need to be hospitalized.

Asthma
Mild intermittent:
- Symptoms ≤ 2 times per week, nighttime symptoms ≤ 2 times per month
- Asymptomatic and normal peak expiratory flow (PEF) between exacerbations
- Exacerbations are brief
- FEV_1 or PEF ≥ 80% predicted, PEF variability < 20%

Mild persistent:
- Symptoms > 2 times per week but < 1 time per day, nighttime symptoms > 2 times per month
- Exacerbations may affect activities
- FEV_1 or PEF ≥ 80% predicted, PEF variability 20% to 30%

Moderate persistent:
- Daily symptoms, nighttime symptoms > 1 time per week
- Daily use of inhaled short-acting β_2-agonist
- Exacerbations affect activity
- Exacerbations ≥ 2 times per week; may last days
- FEV_1 or PEF > 60% to < 80% predicted, PEF variability > 30%

Severe persistent:
- Continual symptoms, frequent nighttime symptoms
- Limited physical activity
- Frequent exacerbations
- FEV_1 or PEF ≤ 60% predicted, PEF variability > 30%

 Provide acute exacerbation treatment if necessary
Short-acting inhaled β_2-selective agonists as needed for symptoms
Usage of short-acting medications more than 2 times per week may indicate that long-term control therapy is necessary.
Oral or parental course of steroids may be indicated if acute exacerbations are severe.

Start Pharmacotherapy
Bronchodilators
- Inhaled β_2-selective agonists (short-/long-acting)
- Oral β-adrenergic agonists
- Anticholinergic agents (ipratropium bromide)
- Theophylline and aminophylline
- Magnesium sulfate

Anti-inflammatory agents
- Glucocorticoids (systemic, oral, or inhaled)
- Cromolyn sodium
- Nedocromil sodium
- Leukotriene inhibitors
- Methotrexate, gold salts, cyclosporine

Educate pt about asthma and develop an action plan for acute exacerbations
Teach correct usage of inhaler and self-monitoring with peak flow meter.
Educate pt about medication roles and proper usage.
Review and update the action plan with each visit.
Refer to support groups.

Discuss environmental control measures
The goal is to avoid or decrease exposure to allergens and irritants.

S **Does the pt present with symptoms of acute bronchitis or pneumonia?**
Pts with bronchitis usually have no or low-grade fever and a normal respiratory rate with diffuse rales.
Pts with pneumonia usually present with fever, dyspnea, tachypnea, and rales over the infected area of lung.

Symptoms are usually gradual in nonbacterial pneumonia and abrupt in bacterial pneumonia.

How long has the pt had the symptoms?
This will help differentiate acute versus chronic bronchitis.

Does the pt have a productive or nonproductive cough?
Bronchitis usually has nonproductive cough early and then progresses into a mucopurulent or productive cough.

Has the pt been exposed to any ill contacts?
Most contagious respiratory infections are caused by viruses.

Is the pt tolerating oral intake?
This will determine if the pt will need IV antibiotics or hydration for infection.

Does the pt have any history of medical problems or comorbidities?
Important comorbidities such as diabetes, asthma, COPD, immune deficiencies, or a history of tobacco, alcohol, or drug abuse may complicate the treatment.
Ascertain if pt has had positive purified protein derivative (PPD) skin test or exposure to tuberculosis.
Review vaccine history for pneumovax and influenza.

Inquire about place of acquisition
Obtaining a history of the pt's recent travels, living, or working environment may be of some assistance in the workup.

 Check vital signs
Look for signs of sepsis or respiratory distress.

Perform physical exam
General: May be ill appearing or unable to speak in full sentences secondary to respiratory distress.
HEENT:
  - Perform exam to rule out upper respiratory infection.
  - Look for grunting or nasal flaring in children.
Lungs: Decreased breath sounds, rales, egophony, tubular breath sounds may be heard, but remember that breath sounds can be normal.
Heart: Perform a complete heart exam.
Skin: Check skin turgor and capillary refill for hydration status.

Consider the following labs and studies:
- CBC	- (PA/LAT CXR)
- Pulse oximetry for O_2 level	- ABG, PaO_2 < 60 warrants admission
- Blood culture if pt appears ill	- Place PPD if suspect TB
- Sputum culture	- Respiratory syncytial virus (RSV) titer if suspected

Bronchitis and Pneumonia
Common bacterial species:

| - *Streptococcus* | - *Haemophilus* | - *Moraxella* |
| *pneumoniae* | *influenzae* | *catarrhalis* |

Atypical species:

| - *Mycoplasma* | - *Chlamydia* | - *Legionella* |
| *pneumoniae* | *pneumoniae* | *pneumophila* |

Viral infections:

| - Rhinovirus | - Influenza virus |
| - Adenovirus | - RSV |

P **Determine severity of illness according to risk factors and clinical presentation**
Risk for mortality should be assessed to determine if pt can be treated as an outpatient or an inpatient.
Risk factors include:
- *If appears ill clinically*   - Age > 65
- WBC < 5000   - Altered mental status
- Suspected *S. aureus*, gram-negative rod, or anaerobic pneumonia
- Metastatic infection such as empyema, meningitis, endocarditis, or arthritis
- Inability to take oral medications
- Comorbid conditions:
  - Renal, cardiac, or pulmonary disease
  - Diabetes, cancer, or immunosuppression
- Signs of severely abnormal physiology:
  - Tachypnea
  - Tachycardia
  - $PaO_2 < 60$
  - Systemic BP < 90 mm Hg

Initiate pharmacotherapy
If it is determined that the pt can be treated as an outpatient, monotherapy with a marcolide is usually first-line treatment. (Fluoroquinolone can also be used.)
Symptomatic relief can be obtained using a cough medication with or without a decongestant.
Antipyretics such as acetaminophen or ibuprofen can be administered for fever or pain.
Consider inhaled bronchodilators if wheezing is present.

Implement prevention
Pneumococcal vaccine
Flu vaccine
Avoidance of tobacco

S **Obtain an abbreviated chest pain history and determine early on if pain is emergent or nonemergent**
If severe chest pain with shortness of breath or diaphoresis presents, then evaluate for cardiac cause.
Determine the severity (0 to 10), character, onset, duration, location, radiation, and alleviating and exacerbating factors of the chest pain.

Does the pt complain of chest pain that suggests cardiac origin?
Typical cardiac pain is described as a substernal pressure-like sensation or tightness with associated radiation to the left arm, neck, jaw, or back.
Chest pain in diabetics may be mild or nonexistent.
Ascertain if there are risk factors for chest pain (e.g., age, male sex, smoker, hypertension, hyperlipidemia, or family history of heart disease).
Pain can be present at rest (unstable angina) or with exertion (stable angina).
Typical cardiac chest pain may resolve or improve with nitrates.

Any gastrointestinal symptoms associated with the chest pain?
Epigastric or burning pain associated with gastritis or ulcers may be mistaken for cardiac pain.
Determine if the pain is related to or relieved by meals, anorexia, or antacids.
Sharp pain localized over the sternum may indicate esophageal spasms.
Dysphagia or odynophagia may cause chest pain.

Is the chest pain reproducible or exacerbated by movement?
Determine if there is repetitive activity, trauma, or injury to the chest wall.
Pain with movement of arms, shoulders, or chest wall may indicate musculoskeletal injury.
Musculoskeletal injuries such as rib fractures can cause chest wall pain with inspiration, at rest, or with movement.

Does the pt have a history of psychological illness?
Panic attacks can present with chest pain along with associated symptoms of shortness of breath, palpitations, dizziness, tremors, tingling, sweating, depersonalization, or feelings of imminent death.
A history of anxiety, depression, or nervousness can point to a psychological cause.

Has the pt had any history of pulmonary problems?
Pulmonary illnesses can present with cough, wheezing, or shortness of breath.
Fever and chills may indicate an infection.

O **Check vital signs**
Determine hemodynamic stability.
Check blood pressure in bilateral arms.

Perform physical exam
General: Observe for signs of anxiety or nervousness.
HEENT: Examine neck for jugular venous distention, carotid pulses, and bruits.
Chest: Perform a complete chest exam; palpate for reproducibility of pain.
Heart: Check rate, rhythm, and auscultate for abnormal heart sounds.
Abdomen: Check for abdominal pain or bruits.
Musculoskeletal: Examine arms, shoulders, and chest wall for tenderness.

Perform the following tests or labs if indicated by history and physical
ECG to rule out cardiac origin of chest pain
Pulse oximetry if shortness of breath
CXR
If epigastric pain is present, consider ultrasound, upper endoscopy, upper
  gastrointestinal series, or barium swallow if indicated.

Chest Pain
Common etiologies include:
- Cardiac causes:
  - Cardiac ischemia   - Congestive heart failure
  - Valvular disease   - Pericarditis
  - Dysrhythmias
- Gastrointestinal causes:
  - Gastritis/gastroesophageal reflux disease
  - Peptic ulcer disease   - Esophageal spasms   - Dyspepsia or flatus
- Musculoskeletal causes:
  - Chest wall muscle strain - Costochondritis (Tietze's syndrome)
  - Upper body trauma or rib fractures
- Psychological causes:
  - Panic attacks   - Generalized anxiety disorder
  - Stress   - Somatization   - Depression
- Pulmonary causes:
  - Pneumonia   - Bronchitis   - Pleurisy
  - Pulmonary embolism   - Pneumothrorax

P Admit pt to hospital if emergent

If cardiac ischemia is suspected, give pt aspirin, oxygen, sublingual nitroglycerin, and
  check ECG.

**If nonemergent, focus treatment on specific cause determined by
history and physical**
Refer to cardiology for a stress test, echocardiogram, or cardiac catheterization.
Remember that myocardial infarction should be ruled out in the hospital.
Appropriate therapy can be started when the diagnosis is made.
See specific topics for treatment

S **Does the pt complain of abdominal pain?**

Detail the pt's abdominal pain.

Pain in acute cholecystitis is described as a sharp, abrupt and severe cramping sensation in the epigastrum or right upper quadrant (RUQ) of the abdomen postprandially.

In chronic disease the pain is gradual, less severe, and without fever.

Nausea, vomiting, and anorexia can accompany the pain.

Cholecystitis may or may not have associated fever and chills.

What types of foods exacerbate or relieve symptoms?

A high-fat diet may exacerbate the disease.

Postprandial pain can be associated with dyspepsia, bloating, or flatus.

Does the pt have risk factors for gallstones?

Risk factors include:

- Obesity	- Female	- Family history
- Childbearing age, but usually 5th decade	- High-fat diet	

Review past medical and surgical history

Determine if there is a history of gastritis, gastroesophageal reflux disease, or peptic ulcer symptoms.

Review symptoms of liver disease such as jaundice, bleeding, or bruising.

O **Check vital signs**

Check for fever and hemodynamic stability.

Perform physical exam

General: Note obesity and if jaundice.

Chest: Auscultate chest for right lower lobe pneumonia.

Abdomen:

- Check for epigastric or RUQ tenderness, rebound, or guarding.
- *Murphy's sign*: Pain in the RUQ that halts inspiration upon palpation
- A palpable gallbladder may indicate cancer.

- *Charcot's triad*: RUQ pain, fever (chills), and jaundice, which may suggest cholangitis.

Consider the following labs:

CBC if cholecystitis is suspected

LFT if jaundice or suspected hepatobiliary disease

Chemistry panel

Amylase if evidence of pancreatitis

Order these tests if indicated

Abdominal ultrasound is the gold standard for diagnosis.

HIDA scan for obstruction of the duct

Abdominal series: Usually not useful unless looking for other causes of pain

CT scan if considering cancer, abscess, or pancreatitis

Cholelithiasis/Cholecystitis
Consider choledocholithiasis and cholangitis if pt is jaundiced.
Consider pancreatitis if pain radiates to the back.

Differential for RUQ abdominal pain may also include:

- Peptic ulcer disease
- Gastritis
- Pericarditis
- Pyelonephritis

- Abdominal cancers
- Liver tumor or abscess
- Pneumonia/pleurisy
- Nephrolithiasis

- Hepatitis
- Myocardial infarction
- Pulmonary embolus

P **Admit if determined the pt has acute cholecystitis**
Keep pt NPO before surgery.
Administer IV fluids.
Start pain management.
Begin IV antibiotic therapy.

Obtain surgical consult for cholecystectomy
Start options for outpatient therapy for cholelithiasis if indicated
Endoscopic retrograde cholangiopancreatography with sphincterotomy may be
indicated if there is a ductal stone or stenosis.
Oral bile salts (ursodiol or chenodiol) can be used in nonsurgical treatment.
Direct solvent dissolution (methyl *tert*-butyl ether or MTBE)
Extracorporeal shock wave lithotripsy

Implement prevention
Exercise, weight management, and low-fat diet

S **Does the pt complain of "pink eye"?**

Conjunctivitis or "pink eye" is caused by inflammation of the conjunctiva.

Associated symptoms can be blurry vision, burning, discharge, photophobia, pain, or excessive tearing.

Is there discharge from the eye?

If discharge is present, determine color and consistency of discharge.

Bacterial conjunctivitis may have thickened exudate with eyelashes glued shut upon awakening.

Viral infections usually have minimal exudate with profuse tearing.

Allergic conjunctivitis typically has severe pruritus with no exudate.

Has the pt had eye trauma?

Eye trauma or foreign objects such as sand, dirt, sawdust, or metal debris can cause inflammation of the conjunctiva and may lead to corneal injuries.

Are there any sick contacts at home, school, or work with "pink eye"?

Infectious conjunctivitis is highly contagious.

Recent upper respiratory infection can precede conjunctivitis.

Is there a history of allergic rhinitis (AR) or asthma that may indicate allergic conjunctivitis?

Associated symptoms of AR are rhinorrhea, nasal congestion, sneezing attacks, and itchiness of the eyes, ears, palate, or throat.

Complaints of wheezing or coughing attacks may be associated with asthma.

Has the pt recently used any products in or around the eye?

New or borrowed eye cosmetics (e.g., eyeliner, mascara, eyeshadow, makeup remover, eye creams, soap, shampoo)

Eye drops or saline solution

Contact lens

 Perform physical exam

HEENT:

- Check pupils' size and reactivity to light.
- Inspect for evidence of photophobia or hyperemia, which may suggest iritis.
- If visual problems are present, examine visual acuity.
- Check for conjunctival discharge, color, and consistency.
- Debris on eyelashes can be seen.
- Inspect for lid edema, vesicles, or allergic shiners (dark circles under eyes).
- Check nares for congestion or mucopurulent discharge.
- Invert eyelids to search for any foreign body.

Consider the following labs or tests:

Fluorescein exam to detect corneal lesions if pt is complaining of pain

Gram stain and culture of discharge if copious

Conjunctivitis
Types:
- Viral conjunctivitis:
  - Most commonly caused by adenoviruses
- Bacterial conjunctivitis:
  - Most commonly caused by *Staphylococcus, Streptococcus,* and *Haemophilus* species
  - If infection seems severe, gonorrhea or chlamydia may be the causative agent.
- Allergic conjunctivitis:
  - Associated with seasonal allergies
  - Exposure to allergens

P After identifying the type of conjunctivitis involved, choose appropriate therapy
Start supportive care for viral conjunctivitis:
- Reassure pt of self-limiting process.
- Emphasize hand washing to limit spread to others.
- Perform daily eye irrigation to remove eyelash debris.
- Decrease rubbing of eye to prevent secondary bacterial infection.
- If herpes is suspected, refer to Ophthalmology immediately.
  - Trifluridine solution may be prescribed.
Start supportive care and topical antibiotics for bacterial conjunctivitis:
- Review interventions listed for viral conjunctivitis.
- Start topical antibiotics in the form of solution drops or ointment.
  - Aminoglycosides
  - Broad-spectrum/polyantimicrobial
  - Quinolone
Start supportive care, topical, and oral medications for allergic conjunctivitis:
- Avoid allergens
- Prescribed medications include:
  - Ocular decongestants
  - Ocular antihistamines
  - Oral antihistamines
  - Ocular mast cell stabilizers

S **How often does the pt defecate per week?**
Normal stooling is three to five times per week, but may vary.
Constipation in children and the elderly can be common.

What are the consistency, color, and shape of the bowel movements?
Pt may complain of smaller or harder stools.
Harder stool may be associated with pain, bleeding, or inadequate bowel evacuation.

Does the pt have inspissated stools?
This may indicate obstruction or impaction.

Any bowel or bladder incontinence?
Incontinence may point to a neurologic deficit or spinal injury.

Does the pt participate in activities or exercise?
A sedentary lifestyle can contribute or exacerbate constipation.

Is the pt taking medication or herbal supplements?
Medications such as opiates, anticholinergics, or iron can cause constipation.
Determine if there is polypharmacy.

Review pt's dietary history
Ascertain pt's intake of fruits, vegetables, fiber, and bran.
Determine pt's daily fluid intake.

Review pt's medical history
Many diseases, such as diabetes and hypothyroidism, can be associated with
  constipation.

Environmental, cultural, psychological, or emotional factors can play a role as well.

O **Perform physical exam**
HEENT:
  • Check for enlarged thyroid gland or goiter.
  • Check for dry mucous membranes or painful oral lesions.
Abdomen:
  • Palpate for masses, tenderness, or distention.
  • Check for hypoactive bowel sounds.
Rectal:
  • Inspect for hemorrhoids, masses, fissures, or impaction.
  • Check sphincter tone, anal wink reflex, and prostate.
  • Guaiac stool
Skin: Check skin turgor, capillary refill, and signs of dry skin.

Consider the following labs if indicated:
CBC to rule out anemia
TSH if thyroid disease is suspected
Chemistry panel for metabolic abnormalities

Order the following radiologic tests if pt does not respond to conservative treatment:
Barium enema or swallow with small bowel follow-through
Colonoscopy or flexible sigmoidoscopy if cancer is suspected or fecal occult blood test
  is positive
KUB to rule out obstruction
Anorectal monometry or biopsy if Hirschsprung's disease is suspected
Timed ingested stool markers to measure transient time

Constipation
Common etiologies:
- Dehydration
- Hypokalemia
- Hypothyroidism
- Psychological disorders
- Uremia in renal failure pt
- Neurologic deficits or injuries

- Poor diet
- Hypercalemia
- Medications, illicit drugs, toxins
- Inactivity
- Diabetic gastroparesis
- Structural causes

Congenital etiologies in children:
- Hirschsprung's disease
- Hypoganglionosis

- Congenital dilation of the colon
- Small left colon syndrome

Treat conservatively unless pt fails treatment or a primary cause is identified
Begin prevention for at-risk populations
Increase or introduce soluble fiber and bran into diet.
Educate pts or parents of pts regarding bowel training.
Discuss importance of hydration.
Increase activity or exercise if pt is sedentary.

Disimpact pt if impacted on rectal exam
Start pharmacotherapy
Bulk-forming agents for primary treatment:
- Methylcellulose (Citrucel)
- Psyllium (Metamucil, Perdiem, Konsyl)
- Barley malt (Maltsupex)
- Calcium polycarbophil (Fibercon, Mitrolan)

Osmotic laxative for short-term use:
- Magnesium citrate
- Milk of magnesia
- Sorbitol
- Phosphate soda
- Glycerin (Fleet)
- Lactulose (Chronulac)
- Polyethylene glycol-electrolyte solution (GoLYTELY)

Irritant cathartics:
- Bisacodyl (Dulcolax)
- Castor oil or ricinoleic acid (Neoloid)

Lubricants: Mineral oil
Surfactants: Docusate sodium (Colace)
Emollient suppositories
Motor and secretory agent: Anthraquinones-senna (Senokot)
Enemas and suppositories with selected agents above

S **Does the pt have long-term or short-term memory loss?**
Obtain a complete symptomatic history from pt, caretaker, nurse, or family.

Are the pt's symptoms abrupt or gradual?

Delirium is a mental impairment of short duration usually caused by a toxic state and can be associated with abnormal attention, fluctuation of consciousness, incoherent speech, disorientation, mental distress, memory impairment, and altered sleep patterns.

Dementia is an organic mental impairment that is gradual and is characterized by loss of intellectual abilities of judgment, memory, abstract thinking, and personality.

Any paranoia, delusions, or hallucinations (visual or auditory)?
These symptoms can coincide with delirium.
Tremor, rigidity, or gait changes can be consistent with Parkinson's disease.

Does the pt have bowel or bladder incontinence?
Pts with incontinence may have a neurologic injury or event.

Is there a history of weight loss or gain?
Pts with dementia often forget to eat and have changes in their weight.

What time of the day does the pt experience the impairment?
Elderly pts can experience more confusion at night.

Does the pt have recent or current history of infection?
Infection is a common cause of delirium in the elderly.

Is there liver or kidney disease producing metabolic disorders?
Review all medications, herbal supplements, and illicit drugs or alcohol use
Side effects from polypharmacy are a problem for pts with multiple illnesses.

Obtain an organ-base review of systems

O **Check vital signs**
Evaluate for signs of infection or sepsis.

Perform physical exam
General: Check if pt is alert and oriented.
HEENT: Search for signs of head trauma.
Chest/Heart: Do a complete cardiopulmonary exam.
Neuro:
- Perform a Mini-Mental Status exam and compare to previous if available.
- Perform a psychological exam and a complete neurologic exam.
- Evaluate for aphasia, agnosia, apraxia, or anomia.

Consider the following labs:
CBC if infection suspected
Chemistry panel for metabolic abnormalities
TSH to rule out thyroid disease
Rapid plasma reagin if evidence of syphilis
Folate/Vitamin B_{12} level
UA or urine culture if UTI suspected
Serum alcohol level
Random serum or urine drug screen
Refer to hospital for lumbar puncture if considering meningitis or encephalitis

Consider these radiologic tests if indicated:
MRI for structural lesions
CT scan if mental impairment is abrupt

 Delirium or Dementia
Common etiologies of delirium:
- Infection   - Metabolic disturbance
- Drugs or toxins   - Hepatic or renal failure
- Thyroid disease   - Hypo-/hyperglycemia
- Head trauma   - Stroke or intracranial hemorrhage
- Hypoxia   - Fecal impaction

Common etiologies of dementia:
- Age-associated dementia   - Alzheimer's/Parkinson's/Huntington's
- Frontotemporal dementia   - Ischemic multi-infarct dementia
- Dementia with Lewy bodies   - Normal pressure hydrocephalus
- Chronic alcoholism   - Postsurgical/anesthesia
- Psychological disorder such as schizophrenia, depression, or elder neglect
- History of central nervous system infection, Down syndrome, or head
  trauma

P **Treatment should be based on the etiology or specific cause of delirium or dementia**
Treat delirium if diagnosed:
- Stop medication or drugs that may cause delirium.
- Admit with close observation, well-lit room and/or restraints.
- Avoid sedation, which may worsen event.

Treat dementia if diagnosed:
- Pt or family can make daily schedules or reminder notes.
- Educate and provide support groups for pt and family.
- Make sure pt's home environment is safe with supervision, and if not, pt may need long-term placement.
- Provide daily stimulation of all senses and encourage socialization.
- Implement medication if behavior treatment fails.

Start pharmacotherapy for specific cause if indicated:
- Levothyroxine replacement for hypothyroidism
- Replacement of vitamin B_{12} and folate if deficient
- Antibiotic treatment for infections
- If psychotic symptoms, antipsychotic medications such as Risperdal, haloperidol, or olanzapine (Zyprexa) can be used.
- Depression or anxiety: See topic (pp. 180 and 186)
- Sleep difficulty: Intermittent use of trazadone (Desyrel), halcion, temazepam (Restoril), zolpidem (Ambien), or chloral hydrate at bedtime
- Donepezil (Aricept) or tacrine (Cognex) can be used for Alzheimer's disease.

S   **Does the pt complain of hypoglycemic or hyperglycemic symptoms?**
Hypoglycemic symptoms include:

- Tremors	- Tachycardia	- Sweating
- Anxiety	- Dizziness	- Hunger
- Weakness	- Fatigue	- Irritability
- Headache	- Blurry vision	

Hyperglycemic symptoms include:

- Drowsiness	- Polyphagia, polydipsia, polyuria
- Dry skin	- Nausea

Any chest pain, shortness of breath, or palpitations?
Diabetics are at increased risk for coronary heart disease (CHD).

Has there been a functional decline in school or work performance?
Absenteeism and functional decline may be related to hypo-/hyperglycemia.

Obtain a complete past medical history and family history
Review history or family history of CHD, hyperlipidemia, or hypertension.
Pts with a history of gestational diabetes have an increased risk of developing diabetes.
Recurrent or slow-healing infections can be associated with diabetes.
If this is the pt's initial visit, consider secondary causes of diabetes such as hemochromatosis, pancreatic disease, or endocrine disorders.

Determine medication adherence
Review diet and daily activities
If known diabetes, review home monitoring values

O   **Check vital signs**
Check fasting or random blood sugar and body mass index.

Perform physical exam
General: Observe body habitus.
HEENT: Perform a funduscopic eye exam to rule out cataracts, retinopathy, or retinal hemorrhage.
Heart: Perform a complete exam to check for abnormalities.
Abdomen: Check for abdominal masses, tenderness, or pain.
Feet: Perform a comprehensive foot exam to check vascular status, skin condition, infections, sensation, and proprioception.
Neuro: Evaluate for peripheral neuropathy.
Skin: Inspect for signs of infections at insulin and fingerstick sites.

Draw the following labs:

- Fasting serum glucose, BUN, and creatinine with chemistry panel
- Hemoglobin A_{1C} (goal < 7)   - UA for glucose, ketones, protein, sediment
- Fasting lipid profile   - Yearly microalbuminuria test

Diabetes Mellitus
Type I:
- Insulin-requiring disease resulting from chronic pancreatic deficiency with inability to produce insulin, leading to end-organ damage from hyperglycemia
Type II:
- Disease that may or may not require insulin, causing hyperglycemia or glucose intolerance secondary to impaired insulin secretion or peripheral action

P **Management is guided by treatment goals set by American Diabetes Association (ADA)**
Start medication to control glucose levels (average preprandial 80–120 mg/dL)
- Biguanide: Metformin (Glucophage)
- Sulfonylureas:
  - First generations: Tolbutamide, tolazamide, chlorpropamide
  - Second generations: Glipizide (Glucotrol), glyburide (Diabeta, Micronase); available in extended release
  - α-glucosidase inhibitor: Acarbose (Precose), miglitol (Glyset)
  - Others: Glimepiride (Amaryl), repaglinide (Prandin), rosiglitazone (Avandia), pioglitazone (Actos)
- Insulins: Regular, NPH, Novulin 70/30, Lente, Ultralente, Lispro, Lantus
Control of blood pressure: See Hypertension (p. 42) for management
- Goal BP is ≤ 130/80
Control dyslipidemia: See Hyperlipidemia (p. 40) for management
- Goal triglycerides < 200 mg/dL and LDL < 100 mg/dL
- Goal HDL > 45 mg/dL in men and > 55 mg/dL in women
Assess complications
- Proteinuria, nephropathy, retinopathy, and neuropathy are common.
Provide preventive therapy and refer when appropriate.
Start dietary and exercise intervention: ADA diet is recommended.
- Recommend mild caloric restriction and mild to moderate exercise.
Adherence of medication and self-care
- Discuss medication compliance and simplify regimen if possible.
- Self-care training with glucose monitoring; exercise, weight, and nutritional management; recognition of signs and symptoms of complications
Follow-up with referrals
- Yearly retinal eye exam by ophthalmologist
- Podiatry for foot and nail care as needed
Immunize pt
- Flu shot yearly
- Tetanus every 10 years
- Pneumococcal vaccine (Pneumovax)

S **What are the pt's symptoms?**
Because dizziness is a vague and subjective symptom, a detailed history is necessary to diagnose the cause.
Obtain the precipitating factors, alleviating factors, frequency, and length of time of the dizziness.
The pt may describe the dizziness as spinning, falling, vertigo, unbalanced, lightheadedness, room spinning, or floor moving.
There can be associated symptoms of headache, numbness, tingling, nausea, or vomiting.

Determine if the dizziness is intermittent or continuous, because continuous may indicate chronic disease.

Is the dizziness consistent with vertigo?
Vertigo is usually described as a sensation of tilting, rotating, or movement of the surroundings.
Vertigo can be associated with an upper respiratory or ear infection.
There may be hearing loss or tinnitus if associated with an ear infection.
Cerebellar or cranial nerve VIII lesions can present with vertigo.
Symptoms can be exacerbated with ambulation or positional changes.

Does the pt complain of near fainting or loss of consciousness?
Presyncopal lightheadedness symptoms can be caused by cardiac disease.
Hypotension or hypovolemia may produce such symptoms.
Symptoms can occur with postural changes, which may indicate vasovagal cause.

Is the pt unsteady with standing or ambulating?
This may indicate a cerebellar problem caused by stroke, transient ischemic attack (TIA), or mass.
These pts will experience an imbalance or disequilibrium.
Obtain any history of brain injury.
Consider peripheral neuropathy if there is a history of diabetes or vitamin deficiency (i.e., folic acid or vitamin B_{12}).
Determine if the pt has a history of multiple sclerosis.

Does the pt have lightheadedness or disoriented dizziness when using eyes?
Ocular-type symptoms can be caused by recent eye surgery or new glasses.
Many diabetic pts with elevated blood sugars can have similar symptoms.
Determine if there has been a loss in visual acuity.

Has the pt felt vague dizziness or derealization?
Obtain a detailed psychological history to rule out depression or anxiety.

Review herbal supplements, illicit drugs, and any medications pt is taking

O **Check vital signs**
Check orthostatic vitals to rule out hypovolemia or orthostatic hypotension.

Perform physical exam
General: May appear ill secondary to nausea and vomiting.

HEENT:
- Determine if there is vertical, horizontal, or rotatory nystagmus.
- Perform a complete ears, nose, throat, and neck exam.

Heart: Examine for arrhythmias or abnormal heart sounds.

Neuro:
- Perform a complete neurologic exam.
- Cerebellar exam: Check gait, Romberg, and finger to nose.
- Hallpike exam to elicite nystagmus or vertigo
- Sensory exam

Consider the following labs and studies if indicated by history:
CBC if signs of infection
Chemistry panel for any electrolyte abnormalities
TSH to rule out thyroid disease
Vitamin B_{12} and folic acid levels for deficiencies
A Snellen and audio test may be indicated.
Holter heart monitor if arrhythmia or palpitation history
Electronystagmography if a vestibular cause is suspected

Radiographic exams
MRI or CT scan to rule out intracranial tumor
Vertebrobasilar Doppler ultrasound if ruling out subclavian steal

Dizziness: *Physical exam and history is key in determining cause*
Vertigo etiologies include:
- Labyrinthitis   - Serous otitis media
- Meniere's disease   - Benign positional vertigo
- TIA or stroke   - Cervical vertigo
- Atypical migraine   - Vesticulopathy

Presyncopal lightheadedness etiologies include:
- Cardiovascular causes   - Postural hypotension
- Vasovagal attacks   - Medication/drugs
- Hypovolemia   - Illness

Imbalance etiologies include:
- Cerebellar lesions   - Multiple sclerosis
- Peripheral neuropathy

Ocular etiologies include:
- Refractive error   - Cataract surgery
- Vision loss   - Hyperglycemia

Other etiologies include: Psychological disorders

If diagnosis is made, treat appropriately
Dizziness symptoms can be reduced with meclizine and antihistamines in vertigo-type illness.
In chronic dizziness secondary to the vestibular symptom, a trial of diazepam may be helpful.
SSRIs or other antidepressants for depression or anxiety
Physical therapy for chronic disease

Refer to a neurologist or specialist if indicated

S **Does the pt complain of urinary symptoms?**
Urinary symptoms can include dysuria, urgency, frequency, hesitancy, nocturia, or
  hematuria.

Any urinary retention, weak stream, or dribbling?
This may indicate prostatic urethral obstruction or enlargement.
Prostatitis can present with rectal or perineal cramping pains.

**Is there a history of urinary tract infection, cystitis, urethritis, or
urethral discharge?**
These infections can easily infect the prostate and epididymis.

Has the pt had pain, swelling, or redness of the testicle?
Testicular pain from the epididymis radiates up the spermatic cord to the inguinal area
  or abdomen.
Usually there is pain with movement or palpation of the testicle.

**Does the pt describe the testicular pain as abrupt with nausea and
vomiting?**
Severe, abrupt pain may indicate torsion and is a medical emergency.

Any myalgias, chills, or fever?
Bacteremia or sepsis can develop in these infections.

**Has the pt had recent urethral instrumentation or Foley catheter
placement?**
Iatrogenic infections during instrumentation may play a major role in diagnosis.

Obtain a sexual history
Ascertain the number of partners, condom use, and type of sex.
Review if the pt or partner has had a sexually transmitted disease (STD).

O **Check vital signs**
Check for fever

Perform physical exam
General: Pt may be ill appearing
Urogenital: Check testicles
  • Testicular or epididymal tenderness with palpation may be present.

  • *Prehn's sign: Reduced testicular pain with elevation of scrotum above symphysis in
    epididymitis (in torsion, there is increased pain)*

  • Examine inguinal lymph nodes.
  • Check for urethral discharge.
  • Evaluate external genitals for lesions.
Rectal: Perform digital rectal exam for enlargement, tenderness, or bogginess of the
  prostate.

Consider the following labs:
UA, urine dip, urine culture
CBC if fever
Blood culture if signs of sepsis
Prostate specific antigen can be elevated in prostatitis
Culture for gonorrhea and chlamydia if suspected
Creatinine if urinary obstruction is suspected

If testicular cause suspected, a testicular ultrasound can be helpful
If torsion is suspected, an inpatient technetium scan can be done

Epididymitis
Usually caused by ascending urethritis
Age > 35 years old, usually enteric organisms such as *Escherichia coli*
Age < 35 years old, consider STD

Prostatitis
Types:
- Acute or chronic bacterial prostatitis
- Nonbacterial prostatitis

Epididymitis treatment
If pt is older than 35 years, treat with a cephalosporin, quinolone, or trimethoprim-
sulfamethoxazole.
If pt is younger than 35 years, treat with ceftriaxone (Rocephin) IM to cover gonorrhea
and doxycycline, ofloxacin, or high-dose macrolide to cover chlamydia.
Pt's partner should be treated if STD is diagnosed.
Provide STD education and counseling.

Acute or chronic bacterial prostatitis treatment
Antibiotic therapy depends on culture results.
If severe, treat with parental antibiotics followed by 4 weeks of oral therapy.
Otherwise, oral treatment should be 4 to 6 weeks long with either a quinolone,
trimethoprim-sulfamethoxazole, or tetracycline.
Symptomatic relief with hydration, pyridium, NSAIDs, and stool softeners
Sitz bath may give some relief.

Nonbacterial prostatitis treatment
Usually does not respond to antibiotics.
Educate pt to avoid alcohol, tobacco, or spicy foods.
Prostatodynia can be treated with an α-adrenergic inhibitor such as prazosin or
terazosin.

Refer to Urology if indicated

S **What are the pt's symptoms?**

Pts with fibromyalgia complain of generalized pain or fatigue.

Fibromyalgia pain can be described as persistent or chronic aching.

The pain can be numbness or burning-type pain.

In order to diagnose this disorder, the pain has to persist for more than 3 months.

This disorder is usually seen in females.

Where does the pt state the pain is located?

Fibromyalgia pain is usually bilateral and located near the neck, back, or joints.

Detail the pt's pain by severity, type, and location.

Are there multiple areas of pain?

Fibromyalgia pain is bilateral or symmetrical in up to 18 paired trigger points.

Is there difficulty awaking or falling asleep?

Obtain a detailed sleep history.

Snoring, daytime sleepiness, and poor sleep hygiene may be consistent with sleep
  apnea, which may be a possible clinical cause of chronic pain.

Does the pt have any medical problems or illnesses?

Several illnesses may be associated with fibromyalgia or have symptoms similar to it
  including:

- Psychological disorders
- Viral or bacterial infections
- Interstitial cystitis
- Irritable bowel syndrome
- Thyroid disease
- Musculoskeletal disease
  (e.g., rheumatoid)
- Temporomandibular joint
  (TMJ) syndrome
- Migraines

O **Check vital signs**
  Perform physical exam

General: May be anxious or have flat affect.

Musculoskeletal: Check for tenderness by digital palpation over 18 paired trigger
  points:

- Bilateral suboccipital muscle insertion
- Bilateral anterior aspect of intertransverse spaces of C5 to C7
- Bilateral trapezius over middle upper border
- Bilateral medial border of the scapular spine
- Bilateral second costochondral junctions
- Bilateral lateral epicondyle
- Bilateral upper lateral gluteal area
- Bilateral posterior greater trochanter
- Bilateral medial fat pad of the knee

Fibromyalgia is a clinical diagnosis and labs are usually normal

Consider the following labs if ruling out other causes of the pt's pain:

CBC if signs of infection

TSH if suspect thyroid disease

Antinuclear antibody for lupus

C-reactive protein to rule out inflammatory disease

Erythrocyte sedimentation rate for inflammation as well

Rheumatoid factor if suspect rheumatoid disease

A sleep study may be done if sleep apnea is suspected

A   **Fibromyalgia is diagnosed by history and physical exam that recognizes pain over 11 of 18 trigger points described above**

P   **Treatment should begin with reassurance**
Start pharmacotherapy
NSAIDs for pain
Tricyclics or SSRIs for depression
Trigger point injection with corticosteroids
Oral corticosteroids have not shown to improve pts' symptoms

Refer to specialists if indicated
Refer to rheumatologist for severe or difficult to treat pts
Physical therapy or exercise program
Refer to psychiatrist or psychologist for therapy
Sleep study if having signs of sleep apnea

Implement prevention
Relaxation techniques and stress management
Proper well-balanced diet

S **What symptoms is the pt experiencing?**

Pts may report symptoms of a burning sensation in the stomach alone (gastritis) or "heartburn" that can be felt in the chest (gastroesophageal reflux disease [GERD]). Laryngitis, hoarseness, shortness of breath, wheezing, nighttime cough, and a bitter taste in the mouth upon awakening can all be caused by GERD.

Are the symptoms worse at any particular time?

In peptic ulcer disease (PUD), symptoms occur on an empty stomach three hours after a meal or at night and are relieved by food.

GERD symptoms usually occur after eating certain foods (see list below), after overeating, and upon recumbency.

Is there any difficulty swallowing (dysphagia) or pain on swallowing (odynophagia)?

Dysphagia can suggest stricture formation of the esophagus from chronic GERD.

Inquire about medical history

Anemia can be secondary to a bleeding peptic ulcer.

Asthma is sometimes precipitated by GERD.

Chest pain caused by GERD can be mistaken for angina.

What medications is the pt taking?

Offending agents may include aspirin, bisphosphonates, NSAIDs, or steroids.

Is there a history of tobacco use?

The risk of developing Barret's esophagitis increases with smoking.

Do certain beverages or foods precipitate the symptoms?

- Alcohol
- Spicy foods
- Peppermint
- Caffeinated beverages: coffee, chocolate, soda, or tea
- Citrus beverages or fruits
- Fatty foods

O **Perform physical exam**

Abdomen:

- Midepigastric tenderness to palpation
- Hyperactive bowel sounds are seen in the setting of a bleeding ulcer
- Peritoneal signs (rebound, guarding, hypoactive bowel sounds) may be elicited when there is gastric perforation from an ulcer.

Rectal: Guaiac positive (bleeding ulcer)

Consider the following labs and studies:

CBC to check for anemia

Helicobacter pylori titers

Amylase and lipase to rule out perforation or pancreatitis

LFT to rule out hepatobiliary disease

ECG to ensure that pain is not cardiac

Upper gastrointestinal series/barium swallow to check for reflux

pH monitoring for 24 hours to assess the degree of acid reflux

Gastritis
Inflammatory changes of the gastric mucosa

Gastroesophageal reflux disease
Damage to esophageal mucosa secondary to reflux of stomach acid and contents

Peptic ulcer disease
Ulceration or mucosal lesion of the stomach or duodenum

Implement lifestyle modifications for all three diseases
- Dietary avoidance   - Smoking/alcohol cessation
- Weight reduction   - Stop/decrease use of offending medications
- Eliminate tight clothing around the waist

Additional lifestyle modifications for GERD
Elevation of the head of bed
Waiting three hours postprandially before recumbency

Initiate pharmacotherapy in a stepwise process
Begin with antacids and over-the-counter H_2 blockers as needed
Step up to daily low-dose H_2 blockers
If little improvement, step up to a high-dose H_2 blocker or proton pump inhibitor
Additional pharmacologic agents for GERD
 • Prokinetic agents
Additional pharmacologic intervention for PUD
 • If *Helicobacter pylori* positive, eradication treatment regimens available:
   ◆ Combinations of antibiotics, H_2 blockers or proton pump inhibitors, and/or bismuth subsalicylate
   ◆ Coating agents: sucralfate or carafate

Refer to Gastroenterology for endoscopy if above interventions fail
Reserve surgical intervention for severe symptoms or complications, including bleeding, obstruction, or perforation
Nissen fundoplication (GERD)
Vagotomy with antrectomy
Vagotomy with pyloroplasty

S **Because of the potential danger of hemorrhage, this is one instance that requires that the pt be assessed before obtaining a detailed history**

Perform quick initial pt assessment and if hemodynamically unstable, insert two large-bore IVs, begin normal saline infusion, and transport to hospital.

If pt is stable, proceed to obtain detailed history of gastrointestinal bleed (GIB)

Hematochezia (bright red blood per rectum) can indicate lower GIB, whereas melena (black, tar-colored stools) typically indicates upper GIB.

Recent fever or diarrhea can suggest an infectious process.

Associated weight loss can be a sign of malignancy.

Bleeding can result from direct abdominal trauma.

Has the pt had recent nosebleeds or vomiting?

Hematemesis (vomiting of blood) that is bright red or the color of coffee grounds can be secondary to blood swallowed from a recent nose bleed or from gastric bleeding.

Violent retching can cause tears that can also lead to hematemesis.

Was there pain associated with the bleed?

External hemorrhoids as opposed to internal ones are typically painful.

Diverticulosis is usually associated with painless bleeding, whereas diverticulitis usually has pain associated in the left lower quadrant.

Ask the pt to quantify the amount of blood lost
What medications is the pt taking?

Offending agents that can lead to GIB are aspirin, bisphosphonates, NSAIDs, and steroids.

Does the pt have a history of heavy alcohol or tobacco use?

Alcohol can lead to liver cirrhosis resulting in portal hypertension and varices.

Tobacco use can lead to peptic ulcers or GI carcinomas.

O **Check vital signs**

Check to see if the pt is hemodynamically stable.

Perform physical exam

General: Pale appearance

HEENT:
- Check for blood in mouth, nares, or oropharynx.
- Inspect for scleral icterus, which can be present in liver disease

Heart: Tachycardia or flow murmur may be audible in high-output states.

Abdomen:
- Inspect for caput medusa, which is typically present in portal hypertension.
- Hyperactive bowel sounds are heard in the setting of bleeding.
- Peritoneal signs (e.g., rebound, guarding, hypoactive bowel sounds) may be elicited when there is perforation.
- Check for ascites, masses, or hepatosplenomegaly.

Rectal: Check for guaiac-positive stool, rectal masses, or hemorrhoids.

Skin: Findings suggesting liver disease include jaundiced skin, palmar erythema, or spider angiomas.

Neuro: Altered mental status may be present in pts who are intoxicated or have elevated ammonia levels (encephalopathy).
- Flapping (asterixis)

Consider the following labs and studies:
CBC to check the hemoglobin level and rule out infection
LFT, prothrombin time/partial thromboplastin time to check for liver disease and coagulopathy
Chemistry panel to check for elevated BUN/creatinine level seen in GIB
Radiologic imaging, such as x-ray, ultrasound, or CT scan, may be needed.

Gastrointestinal bleed
Types delineated anatomically in relation to the ligament of Treitz
- Upper GIBs (above the ligament) are caused by:
    - Arteriovenous malformations
    - Erosive gastritis
    - Mallory-Weiss tear
    - Duodenal/gastric ulcer
    - Esophagitis
    - Varices
- Lower GIBs (below the ligament) are caused by:
    - Angiodysplasia
    - Cancer
    - Diverticulosis
    - Anorectal hemorrhoids
    - Colitis
    - Polyps

Upper GI bleed management
Place nasogastric tube to aspirate stomach contents: Bloody return indicates upper GIB and admission to the hospital.
- Place on NPO restrictions.
- Obtain serial CBCs to assess if pt is actively bleeding.
- Start IV proton pump inhibitor or H_2 blocker empirically.

Treat as an outpatient if the pt has no active bleeding, a stable hemoglobin, and is not orthostatic.
Obtain a GI consult for upper endoscopy.
- May require banding, balloon tamponade, sclerotherapy, transjugular intrahepatic portosystemic shunt (TIPS), or surgery if bleeding continues.

Lower GI bleed management
After upper GI bleed is excluded via negative nasogastric aspiration, pt remains NPO, and proceeds with lower gastrointestinal workup as inpatient.
If the pt is stable, as above, treat as an outpatient.
Consult GI specialist for possible anoscopy, sigmoidoscopy, or colonoscopy.
Order a tagged red blood cell nuclear scan if no source is found and there is still active bleeding.
Obtain a surgical consult if bleeding persists or is life threatening.

S

What quality of pain does the pt describe?
Cluster headaches are described as stabbing pains usually located behind one eye.
Tension headaches are reported as tight, squeezing pressures.
Throbbing or pulsating pains are typical of migraine headaches.

What triggers headaches?
Migraines can be triggered by menses, strong odors, lack of sleep, and hypoglycemia.
Stress is the primary trigger of tension headaches.

Are there symptoms accompanying the headache?
Scalp tenderness, jaw claudication, sudden loss of vision, weight loss, and polymyalgia
  rheumatica can be present in giant cell arteritis (temporal arteritis).
Cluster headaches can have lacrimation and ptosis.
Migraine headaches can be accompanied by an aura of scintillating light, nausea,
  vomiting, phonophobia, or photophobia.
New-onset seizures can be a sign of increased intracranial pressure (tumor).

Has the pt tried any medications for the headaches in the past?
Gather information regarding treatment failures, successes, and satisfaction.

Obtain medical history
A history of cancer, collagen-vascular disease, diabetes, glaucoma, hypertension, or
  sinusitis can be linked to headaches.

**Is the pt taking any medications, natural herbs, supplements, or
vitamins?**
  - Oral contraceptive   - Narcotics   - Nitrates
  - Sildenafil   - Vitamin A

Any recent trauma?
A concussion, fall, or recent lumbar puncture can precede headaches.

Is there a family history of headaches?
Cluster and migraine headaches are known to have a genetic predisposition.

O

Check vital signs
Check for fever or elevated blood pressure.

Perform physical exam
HEENT:
  • Check head for lacerations
  • Hemotympanum, mastoid bruising (Battle's sign), raccoon eyes, and clear
    otorrhea or rhinorrhea suggest a basilar skull fracture.
  • Scalp or temporal tenderness can be present in giant cell arteritis tenderness.
  • Unequal pupils are seen in cluster headaches and in increased intracranial
    pressure.
  • Papilledema on funduscopy is a finding with increased intracranial pressure.
  • Temporomandibular joint (TMJ) tenderness and "Z"-shaped jaw opening are
    present in TMJ disease.
  • Check for rigidity, which can be present in meningitis.
Neuro:
  • Check all cranial nerves; test visual fields, motor, and sensory exams.
  • Check for cerebellar deficits: alternating hands, finger-to-nose, and gait.

Consider the following labs and studies:
ESR can be elevated in giant cell arteritis.
Imaging via CT scan or MRI to rule out intracranial bleed, fracture, or tumor
Lumbar puncture: Gram stain, cell count, VDRL, culture and sensitivities

 Headache
Primary types:
- *Cluster*: Centered around one or both orbits; associated red, tearing eye, miosis, ptosis, and rhinorrhea
- *Migraine*: Unilateral, with or without aura, described as throbbing; associated nausea, vomiting, phonophobia, photophobia; aggravated by activity
- *Tension*: Bilateral band-like pressure not aggravated by activity

Secondary types:
- *Giant cell arteritis*: Scalp tenderness, jaw pain, and visual changes can be associated
- *Meningitis*: Caused by a bacterial/viral infection with nuchal rigidity and fever
- *Subarachnoid hemorrhage*: Described as the worst headache ever with sudden onset

Other secondary causes
- Altitude
- Herpes zoster
- Tumors
- Hypo-/hyperglycemia
- Sinusitis
- Glaucoma
- TMJ disease

P Treat primary headaches
Educate pt about disease and suggest behavioral changes:
- Adopt regular patterns of sleeping, eating, exercise, and stress reduction.
- Address psychosocial issues.

Start medications to reduce frequency and severity of headaches and improve quality of life:
- NSAIDs
- Combination analgesics
- Ergotamines
- Narcotics (limited use is recommended)
- Tryptans (for migraines)

Initiate preventive therapy for headache prophylaxis:
- Anticonvulsants
- Antihypertensives
- Antidepressants

Refer to Neurology if treatment fails or pain escalates.

Treat secondary headaches based on the primary cause
Admit pts with the following:
- *Giant cell arteritis*: Temporal artery biopsy, initiation of steroids, serial ESRs
- *Meningitis*: Lumbar puncture, empiric antibiotics, and/or antivirals until culture results are obtained
- *Subarachnoid hemorrhage*: Neurosurgery consult, blood pressure control, and anticonvulsants

S **Does the pt have a history of hyperlipidemia?**
Because hyperlipidemia usually does not cause symptoms, it is important that
associated disease symptoms be assessed.
Ascertain if there are symptoms that may indicate cardiac or neurologic disease.

Is there a history of illness that may cause hyperlipidemia?
Common diseases that may cause hyperlipidemia are hypothyroidism, diabetes,
obesity, chronic renal failure, and nephrotic syndrome.
Alcohol abuse or anabolic steroid use can also cause hyperlipidemia.
Assess history of coronary heart disease (CHD) or CHD-equivalent diseases such as
stroke, transient ischemic attack (TIA), peripheral vascular disease, and abdominal
aortic aneurysm.

Does the pt have a family history of hyperlipidemia?
Xanthomas and premature CHD may indicate a familial dyslipidemia.

Does the pt smoke?
Smoking history is important when assessing risk for CHD.

Review pt's diet and exercise routine

O **Perform physical exam**
Neck: Check for carotid bruits and pulses.
Heart: Perform a complete heart exam.
Abdomen: Listen for renal bruits.
Neuro: Perform a complete neurologic exam if signs of stroke or TIA are present.
Skin: Look for xanthomas near eyelids or over extensor areas of tendons.

Obtain a complete fasting lipid profile
- Total cholesterol   - Low-density lipoprotein (LDL)
- Triglycerides   - High-density lipoprotein (HDL)

A **Hyperlipidemia**
Assess risk factors, including:
- Tobacco use   - Age (Men $\geq$ 45 y/o or women $\geq$ 55 y/o)
- Hypertension   - Family history of premature CHD
- Low HDL < 45 mg/dL   - If HDL > 60 mg/dL, subtract one risk factor
- If pt has two or more risk factors, calculate 10-year CHD risk using the
Framingham scoring system (see www.nhlbi.nih.gov/about/framingham/
index.html).
This global assessment determines treatment guidelines for the target LDL.

P **Implement diet, weight management, and exercise as first-line
treatment**
Dietary recommendations:
- Reduce saturated fat to < 7% of total cholesterol
- Reduce cholesterol intake to < 200 mg daily
- Increase plant stanols or sterols to 2 g daily
- Increase soluble fiber to 10–23 g daily

Optimize modifiable risk factors
CHD risk factors, such as age, sex, and family history cannot be modified, but diabetes,
hypertension, smoking, hyperlipidemia, and obesity can.

Initiate pharmacotherapy if diet therapy fails after 12 weeks

3-hydroxy-3-methylglutaryl-coenzyme A reductase inhibitors or statins

- Fluvastatin sodium
- Simvastatin
- Lovastatin
- Pravastatin sodium
- Atorvastatin
- Rosuvastatin

Fibrates

- Gemfibrozil
- Fenofibrate

Bile acid sequestrants

- Colestipol
- Cholestyramine
- Colesevelam

B-complex vitamin

- Niacin

Cholesterol absorption inhibitor

- Ezetimibe

Treatment goals are separated into three categories to reduce cardiovascular risk:

Coronary heart disease or risk equivalent (10-year risk > 20%):

- LDL goal < 100 mg/dL
- Lifestyle changes if LDL ≥ 100 mg/dL
- Pharmacotherapy if LDL ≥ 130 mg/dL (optional if 100–129 mg/dL)

Two or more risk factors (10-year risk ≤ 20%):

- LDL goal < 130 mg/dL
- Lifestyle changes if LDL ≥ 130 mg/dL
- Pharmacotherapy if LDL ≥ 130 mg/dL and 10-year risk 10% to 20%
- Pharmacotherapy if LDL ≥ 160 mg/dL and 10-year risk < 10%

Zero or one risk factor:

- LDL goal < 160 mg/dL
- Lifestyle changes if LDL ≥ 160 mg/dL
- Pharmacotherapy if LDL ≥ 190 mg/dL
- Pharmacotherapy is optional if LDL = 160–190 mg/dL

More aggressive combination therapy should be introduced if pt has a low HDL < 40 mg/dL with a triglyceride level > 200 mg/dL or other mixed dyslipidemias

Combination therapy along with fish oil for severely elevated triglycerides

Screening

All adults 20 years of age or older should be screened every five years.
Test earlier if there is a family history or pt is obese.

S **Does the pt complain of headaches or visual symptoms?**

Hypertension can present with visual disturbances and headaches.

Visual disturbances can be caused by late complications, such as retinal exudates, vascular narrowing, hemorrhages, or retinopathy.

Are there cardiac symptoms such as chest pain, palpitations, or syncope?

Hypertension can initially present with cardiac symptoms; however, pt is usually asymptomatic.

If pt has associated coronary heart disease (CHD), obtain a history of pulmonary symptoms, such as cough, shortness of breath, paroxysmal nocturnal dyspnea, or dyspnea on exertion.

Any neurologic deficits or motor weakness?

Pts with long-standing hypertension can present with transient ischemic attack (TIA) or stroke.

Review pt's diet, medications, substance use, and activities

Topics to review include illicit drug use, alcohol abuse, smoking, medications, diet (including sodium intake), and herbal or nutritional supplements.

Does the pt or family have a history of hypertension or related illnesses?

Pts with hypertension can have related heart disease, diabetes, renal disease, peripheral vascular disease, or hyperlipidemia.

Hypertension has a strong genetic disposition.

O **Check vital signs**

Measure BP in both arms to rule out coarctation or dissection of the aorta.

Perform physical exam

HEENT:

- Check for jugular venous distention (JVD), carotid bruits, and pulses.
- Perform a (dilated) funduscopic exam for papilledema, retinal exudates, hemorrhages, or retinopathy.

Chest: Auscultate for abnormal lung sounds, such wheezing, crackles, or rales.

Heart: Check for arrhythmias, S3, S4, murmurs, or a displaced point of maximal impulse (PMI).

Abdomen: Listen for renal bruits and palpate for masses or pain.

Neuro: Perform a complete neurologic exam for signs of stroke or TIA.

Consider the following labs:

CBC with differential

Chemistry panel for electrolyte abnormalities

RUDS if suspected drug use

UA for proteinuria

Urine metanephrines if pheochromocytoma is suspected

Consider these tests if indicated:

ECG for baseline or for acute chest pain

CXR to rule out cardiomegaly or pulmonary congestion

Two-dimensional echocardiogram if left ventricular dysfunction is suspected or audible murmur

CT scan or MRI of the head if neurologic deficits present
CT scan of the abdomen if suspect aortic dissection or pheochromocytoma
Renal ultrasound if considering renal artery stenosis

 Hypertension: Stage according to the Joint National Committee (JNC) on Prevention, Detection, Evaluation, and Treatment of High Blood Pressure VII Report
Prehypertension: 120–139/80–89 mm Hg
Stage 1: 140–159/90–99 mm Hg
Stage 2: ≥ 160/≥ 100 mm Hg

 Treat according to the strategies recommended in the JNC-VII
Prehypertension: Treat with lifestyle modifications of diet, exercise, and weight reduction.
Stage 1: Treat with monotherapy but consider coexisting conditions.
  • Thiazide diuretics are the first-line treatment for hypertension, followed by β-blockers, angiotensin-converting enzyme (ACE) inhibitors, and calcium channel blockers.
Stage 2: Treat with two-drug therapy that should be tailored to pt's coexisting conditions.
  • Combination therapy usually with a thiazide diuretic and either a β-blocker or ACE inhibitor can be implemented.

Implement the Dietary Approaches to Stop Hypertension (DASH) diet
Vegetables, fruit, whole grains, nuts, fish, poultry, and low-fat diary products
This diet is high in magnesium, potassium, and calcium but low in sodium
Pts with diabetes and chronic kidney disease should be treated with pharmacotherapy

Optimize blood pressure goals
Isolated systolic hypertension goal < 140 mm Hg
Diabetes or chronic renal disease goal is ≤ 130/80 mm Hg

Individualize treatment according to comorbidities
Diabetics can be started on ACE inhibitors, angiotensin-II receptor blockers (ARBs), thiazide diuretics, or β-blockers.
ACE inhibitors or ARBs should be used in diabetes or chronic renal insufficiency to prevent worsening cardiovascular or renal disease.
Pts with cardiovascular disease should be started on β-blockers and an ACE inhibitor.
If cough develops with an ACE inhibitor, an ARB can be used to replace the ACE inhibitor.
Nondihydropyridine calcium channel blockers can be used in pts with diastolic dysfunction heart failure, angina, or superventricular tachycardia.
The newest class of medicines are the selective aldosterone receptor antagonists, which are indicated as adjunct therapy in pts with heart failure.

S **What symptoms is the pt reporting?**
Pts usually describe vasomotor symptoms of hot flushes, heat intolerance, and
  increased sweating.
Nervousness, palpitations, or tremulousness can suggest arrhythmia.
Complaints of fatigue, weakness, and insomnia are typical in hyperthyroidism.
Despite increase in appetite, pts experience weight loss.
Difficulty concentrating, irritability, and emotional instability may be reported.

Is the pt experiencing gastrointestinal changes?
Frequent bowel movements and greasy stools (steatorrhea) are common.

If female, has there been a change in her menstrual cycle?
Recent changes of irregularity such as oligomenorrhea or amenorrhea occur with
  hyperthyroidism.

Review current medications or supplements
Pts taking any weight loss pills may inadvertently be ingesting exogenous thyroid
  hormone.

Do any family members have thyroid problems?
There is a genetic predisposition in hyperthyroidism.

Has the pt noticed any changes in vision?
Exophthalmos and proptosis can lead to optic nerve atrophy and corneal abrasions.

O **Perform physical exam**
General: Restlessness may be observed.
HEENT:
- Diplopia, lid lag, or proptosis
- Tongue tremor or fasciculations can be observed.
- Enlargement of thyroid or palpable nodules can be found.
- Auscultate the thyroid gland for bruits.
Heart:
- Hyperdynamic chest or flow murmur may be present.
- An irregular rate suggests atrial fibrillation.
Skin:
- Moist, warm, silky skin along with fine, silky hair are common findings.
- Check for fingernail separation from nail bed (onycholysis).
Neuro:
- Elicit deep tendon reflexes, which are usually brisk in hyperthyroidism.
- Inspect hands for fine tremor.

Consider the following labs and studies:
Thyroid-stimulating hormone (TSH) is low, whereas free T4 is elevated.
Occasionally will need T3 (if TSH is low and free T4 is normal)

Thyroid-stimulating immunoglobulins (TSIs) mimic TSH and increase thyroid
  activity in Graves' disease

ECG to record tachyarrhythmia
Technetium-99 thyroid scan:
- Low uptake suggests thyroiditis or hormone use.
- High uptake suggests Graves' disease or toxic nodule(s).

A **Hyperthyroidism**
Common causes:
- Autoimmune: Referred to as Graves' disease
- Autonomous thyroid nodule(s):
    - Thyroid adenoma
    - Toxic multinodular goiter
- Iatrogenic or factitious: Caused by the use of exogenous thyroid hormone

Less common causes:
- TSH or TSH-like secreting tumor:
    - Pituitary adenoma
    - Hydatidiform mole or choriocarcinoma (via human chorionic gonadotropin)
- Ectopic hormone production: Ovarian teratoma (struma ovarii)

P **Consider the following therapeutic options**
Start medications.
- β-blockers: Used to control the symptoms of anxiety, palpitations, and tremor.
- Antithyroid drugs: Inhibit thyroid hormone synthesis
    - Methimazole
    - Propylthiouracil

Refer to Endocrinology for consideration of radioactive iodine.
- Used to ablate thyroid tissue

Refer to Surgery.
- Subtotal thyroidectomy is reserved for those who fail antithyroid drugs, have severe disease, or large goiters.
- Pts with pituitary adenoma, hydatidiform mole, choriocarcinoma, or ovarian teratoma need appropriate referrals as well.

Additional considerations
Refer to Ophthalmology if exophthalmos is present.

S **What symptoms has the pt noticed?**

Pts report cold intolerance, fatigue, lethargy, weakness, and hair loss.

Additionally, they may notice that despite a decreased appetite, there is weight gain.

Gastrointestinal problems arise from a decreased frequency of bowel movements, which leads to constipation.

Galactorrhea can suggest a problem with hypothyroidism.

Does the pt have any autoimmune disorders?

Diseases that increase the risk of hypothyroidism include:

- Addison's disease   - Diabetes mellitus
- Pernicious anemia   - Systemic lupus erythematosus
- Sjögren   - Rheumatoid arthritis
- Vitiligo

Does the pt have a problem with hyperlipidemia?

Elevation in cholesterol is a common finding.

Has the pt had hyperthyroidism in the past?

Prior radioactive iodine treatment, neck irradiation, or thyroid surgery can result in hypothyroidism.

Any family history of thyroid disease?
Review current medications

Medications known to influence thyroid function include α-interferon, lithium, and amiodarone.

If female, ask about menstruation

Pts may experience heavy menses (menorrhagia).

Hemorrhage at time of delivery predisposes pt to panhypopituitarism (Sheehan's syndrome).

 Perform physical exam

General: Pt may be expressionless with slow speech.

HEENT:

- Check for periorbital puffiness or loss of lateral third of eyebrows.
- Palpate the thyroid for possible goiter.

Heart:

- Auscultation may reveal bradycardia with muffled heart sounds, suggesting pericardial effusion.
- The point of maximal impulse (PMI) can be displaced, indicating an enlarged heart.

Chest: Nipple discharge can be present on breast exam.

Abdomen: Decreased or absent bowel sounds on auscultation secondary to ileus

Neuro: Delayed relaxation of deep tendon reflexes is elicited.

Skin:

- Rough, cool skin, with a doughy consistency
- Orange-yellow coloration
- Nonpitting pretibial edema (myxedema)
- Brittle hair and nails, pitting of the fingernails

Consider the following labs and studies:

Thyroid-stimulating hormone (TSH) is high, whereas free T4 is low.

Thyroid receptor-blocking antibodies suggest Hashimoto's disease.

ECG to check that there is no heart block or bradycardia

Lipid panel

Hypothyroidism
Common causes:
- Autoimmune: Referred to as Hashimoto's thyroiditis
- Iatrogenic:
  - Status post-treatment of hyperthyroidism
    - After administration of radioactive iodine
    - After surgical resection of thyroid
  - Secondary to the use of medications
    - See medications listed in "S" section

Other causes:
- Iodine deficiency: Not common because salt is now iodized
- Eternal radiation therapy
- Panhypopituitarism:
  - Referred to as Sheehan's syndrome (postpartum hemorrhage)

P **Starting hormone replacement pharmacotherapy with thyroxine**
Many different preparations are available.

Check serial serum TSH
Must draw laboratory every 4 to 6 weeks after making adjustments to thyroxine.

Supplement iodine
Only used if deficiency is the cause for hypothyroidism.

S **What symptoms suggesting nephrolithiasis does the pt express?**
Symptoms of sudden, intense flank or abdominal pain that are associated with nausea,
    vomiting, or fever can be present with nephrolithiasis.
Blood in the urine (hematuria) can indicate nephrolithiasis.
Pts can have a decrease in urine production if obstruction is severe.

Does the pt have irritative urinary symptoms?
Typically, the pt reports frequency, urgency, and burning pain (dysuria) with urination.
A history of multiple UTIs warrants an investigation for nephrolithiasis.
Changes in urine volume: Decreased amount of urine production can be present.

Does the pt have radiation of the pain?
Usual route of the stone as it traverses the urogenital system: back, flank, lower
    abdomen, groin, or vulva

Has the pt had any prior episodes of nephrolithiasis?
Pts with a history of gout or hyperparathyroidism are prone to stone formation
    secondary to a high level of uric acid and calcium.

O **Check vital signs**
Fever can be a sign of urine infection.

Perform physical exam
General: Pt may be in writhing pain, unable to find a comfortable position.
Abdomen:
  • Bowel sounds may be normal or decreased.
  • Tenderness may be present on palpation in suprapubic and/or renal areas.
Back: Costovertebral angle tenderness (CVAT) may be unilateral or bilateral, suggesting
    pyelonephritis.
Urogenital/Pelvic:
  • If male, check for hernias, testicular/scrotal masses, or epididymal tenderness,
    which could be mimicking nephrolithiasis.
  • If female, check for cervical motion tenderness, vaginitis, adnexal masses, or
    tenderness, which could be mimicking nephrolithiasis.

Consider the following labs and studies:
UA: Leukocyte esterase and nitrites are positive in infection.
  • Gross or microscopic blood suggests nephrolithiasis.
Chemistry panel: Creatinine may be elevated secondary to obstruction.
Urine culture if UA dip suggests infection
KUB: Most stones are radiopaque.
Intravenous pyelogram versus spiral CT scan:
  • Both can reveal the site of obstruction (proximal versus distal).
  • Both can detect the presence of hydonephrosis.
Renal ultrasound versus CT scan:
  • Both can detect perinephric abscess.

A **Nephrolithiasis**
Types of calculi:
- Calcium oxalate   - Cystine
- Struvite   - Uric acid

P **Treat as an outpatient:**
Medications for pain: NSAIDs and opiates
Treat with oral or intramuscular antibiotics if infection is suggested.
Instruct pt to strain all urine voids in attempts to retrieve the calculus.
Send calculus for analysis to determine its composition.
Counsel pts regarding avoidance of dehydration and fluid loading in all types of
  nephrolithiasis.

Hospitalize pt if calculus does not pass, pain persists for longer than two days, or fever
  develops.

Treat calcium oxalate stones with:
Thiazide diuretics

Treat cystine stones with:
Low salt and protein diet
Alkali supplements (potassium citrate, Shohl's solution)

Treat struvite stones with:
pH-lowering agents (methenamine, acetohydroxamic acid)
Refer to Urology.

Treat uric acid stones with:
Low purine diet
Allopurinol
Alkali supplements (see above)

Refer for further interventions if calculus does not pass:
Urology:
  • Extracorporeal shock wave lithotripsy
  • Nephrostomy or stent placement

S **Has the pt always had a weight problem or just recently?**
Many children or adolescents who are obese will continue with the same problem into adulthood.
It is important to find out what measures the pt has taken to lose weight.

What are the pt's triggers for eating?
Some pts report insatiable appetite, depression, or stress as triggers.

Does the pt have scheduled mealtimes?
Pts with erratic or busy schedules will skip meals, snack throughout the day, eat at fast-food restaurants, and eat late meals.

Does the pt have any risk factors for coronary heart disease (CHD)?
- Diabetes mellitus   - Hyperlipidemia
- Family history of CHD   - Hypertension
- Sedentary lifestyle   - Tobacco use

Has the pt had health conditions associated with obesity?
Amenorrhea/menorrhagia, osteoarthritis, obstructive sleep apnea, stress incontinence, back/large joint pain requiring surgical intervention or replacement can all arise from obesity.

Review medications the pt is taking
Drugs known to cause weight gain include:
- Antidepressants   - Depakote
- Insulin   - Lithium
- Steroids   - Oral contraceptives

Is the pt currently involved in an exercise program?

Increasing daily physical activity is a cornerstone to weight loss.

O **Check vital signs**
Check for hypertension
Determine body mass index (BMI)

Perform physical exam
General: Observe for central obesity.
HEENT: Check thyroid for enlargement.
Abdomen: Measure waist circumference and palpate for masses.
Skeletal: Joint crepitus, tenderness, or deformity may be present.

Consider the following lab and studies:
Fasting glucose to rule out diabetes mellitus or glucose intolerance
TSH to rule out thyroid disease
Fasting lipid panel to assess for dyslipidemia

Obesity is classified using BMI

BMI is a calculation incorporating the height and weight of an individual to yield the classification of obesity.

The higher the classification, the higher the potential health risk.

Formula for BMI: weight (kg)/height(m^2)

- Class I: BMI of 30.0–34.9
- Class II: BMI of 35.0–39.9
- Class III: BMI ≥ 40 considered extreme or morbid obesity

Metabolic syndrome can be diagnosed if at least three criteria are met:

Central obesity:

- Men with waist circumference > 102 cm (40 inches)
- Women with waist circumference > 88 cm (35 inches)

Hypertriglyceridemia: ≥ 150 mg/dL

Low HDL:

- Men < 40 mg/dL
- Women < 50 mg/dL

Hypertension: ≥ 130/85 mm Hg

Fasting glucose impairment: ≥ 110 mg/dL

P **Behavioral strategies must incorporate diet and exercise**

Initiate goal to promote fitness:

- Begin the shift from a sedentary to active lifestyle to prevent weight gain.
  - ◆ Establish regular exercise: 3 to 5 times per week.
  - ◆ Gradually increase duration and intensity.
- Once weight gain ceases, set realistic goals for weight loss.

Review food pyramid, emphasizing a low-fat, low-calorie diet and portion control.

Establish scheduled meal times: No late-night meals or snacks.

Start pharmacotherapy

Medications for appetite suppression: fenfluramine and sibutramine

Medication for fat-binding/lipase inhibition: orlistat

Consider referrals

Consult nutritionist to direct the pt on how to combine balanced meal plans and to provide assistance in identifying and correcting poor dietary choices.

Surgeon

- Surgical interventions aimed at manipulating absorption include:
  - ◆ Gastric bypass
  - ◆ Gastroplasty
  - ◆ Gastric banding

S **Does the pt have risk factors for osteoarthritis?**

- Age > 50 years   - History of immobilization
- Obesity   - Joint hypermobility/instability
- Peripheral neuropathy   - Injury/trauma to the joint
- Crystals in joint fluid   - Prolonged occupational/sports stress

When is the pain worse?

Pts with osteoarthritis (OA) perceive pain with stiffness upon awakening or after
prolonged rest.
Movement usually alleviates the pain in 30 minutes.

What joints are involved?

Affected joints usually involve distal interphalangeal (DIP), proximal interphalangeal
(PIP), first carpometacarpal, knee, hip, cervical spine, and lumbosacral spine.
The joint pain is usually gradual over time.

Is the pt having any systemic symptoms?

Consider inflammatory arthritides if fever, weight loss, nail changes, skin rashes, or
ocular symptoms are present: rheumatoid arthritis, systemic lupus erythematosus,
Sjögren's syndrome, Reiter's syndrome, psoriatic arthritis.

O **Perform physical exam**

Musculoskeletal:

- Joints can have decreased range of motion measured in degrees.
- Herberden's nodes can be present on the DIP joints.
- Bouchard's nodes can be present in the PIP joints.
- Joint deformities or enlargements may be observed.
- Pain with movement or tenderness over the joint margins may be elicited with palpation.
- Inspect for local trauma, erythema, or streaks, suggesting a septic arthritis.
- Crepitus and joint instability are late signs in osteoarthritis
- Synovitis or effusion may be present

Labs are usually not useful, and diagnosis is based on clinical exam and x-rays

Joint aspiration can be used to differentiate OA from inflammatory arthritis:

- < 500 WBCs/mL in OA with monocyte predominance
- > 2000 WBCs/mL in inflammatory arthritis with neutrophil predominance

Erythrocyte sedimentation rate is usually normal or slightly elevated in OA, markedly
elevated in rheumatoid.
X-rays are normal early on, and later there is narrowed joint space, subchondral bony
sclerosis, osteophytes (spurs), subchondral cysts, erosions, and osseous bodies in the
joint space.

A **Osteoarthritis**
OA is a progressive degenerative joint disease, and diagnosis is based on history, clinical findings, and radiographic films.

P **The treatment goals for OA are to reduce pain, improve or maintain function, and prevent or slow progression**
Recommend conservative interventions
Weight loss if obese
Reduce overuse of joints
Heat and ice therapy
Capsaicin cream
Assess functional status and provide mobility aids such as canes, walkers, etc.
Physical therapy to increase function and strength
Pt education and support groups can be useful (Arthritis Foundation).

Start pharmacotherapy
Acetaminophen is recommended if pt has a history of peptic ulcer disease.
Nonacetylated salicylates
NSAIDs
Newer NSAIDs
- Cox-2 inhibitors have decreased risk of ulcers.
Opioid analgesics can be used for severe pain.
Joint injections with steroids to reduce acute inflammation (3 to 4 per joint per year)

Consider alternative therapies
Hyaluronic acid injections into the affected joint (series of three injections)
        - Sodium hyaluronate (Hyalgan)   - Hylan G-F 20 (Synvisc)
Proteoglycan substance has been shown to have mild anti-inflammatory effects on the articular cartilage.
- Glucosamine sulfate 1500 mg/day
- Chondroitin sulfate 1200 mg/day

Refer to orthopedic surgeon
Surgical interventions may be indicated in pts with severe functional decline and intractable pain:
- Athroscopic lavage and extraction of loose bodies
- Debridement
- Osteotomy
- Total joint replacement

S

What types of symptoms is the pt reporting?
Symptoms may include scratchy or sore throat, dysphagia, fever, headaches, cough, rhinorrhea, myalgias, nasal congestion, rash, and conjunctivitis.
Pts will sometimes complain of referred pain to the ear.
A strawberry tongue can appear in group A streptococcal infections.

Does the pt have a history of recurrent throat infections?
Pts exposed to sick contacts (e.g., in daycare facilities) can have recurrent infections.
Symptoms of allergic rhinitis can be mistaken for throat infections.
Tonsillectomy may be indicated if pt experiences two to three episodes of documented streptococcal pharyngitis infections within 6 months.

Does the pt report any recent skin rashes?
Viral exanthems can erupt 48 to 72 hours after sore throat begins.

Scarlet fever exanthem described as "sandpaper rash" starts on the upper trunk, spreads throughout the body, and spares the perioral area (perioral pallor).

Has the pt's voice changed?
Loss of voice (laryngitis) is typically caused by viral infections.
"Hot-potato voice" can be a sign of peritonsillar swelling.

Is the pt sexually active?
Performing oral sex without a protective barrier places the pt at risk for pharyngeal infection with gonorrhea.

O

Check vital signs
Check for fever.

Perform physical exam
HEENT:
- Palatal petechiae, beefy red tonsillar appearance, exudates, and a strawberry tongue can all be findings of streptococcal infection.
- Presence of nasal congestion, clear rhinorrhea, and erythematous oropharynx can be seen in viral pharyngitis.
- Vesicles or ulcerations on the oral mucosa can be present in herpes and coxsackie infections.
- Unilateral soft palate swelling with displacement of uvula is evident in peritonsillar abscess.

Neck:
- Check for cervical adenitis.
- Auscultate to check for stridor, which can be present in *Haemophilus influenzae*.

Skin:
- Inspect for the presence of a "sandpaper rash," which arises from the toxin of group A streptococcal infection.
- Linear petechiae on the body folds of the neck, groin, axilla, antecubital fossa, and popliteal fossa called "Pastia's lines" can also be found in scarlet fever.
- Inspect palms and soles for vesicles when coxsackie infection is suspected.

Consider the following labs and studies:
Rapid strep assay: If negative, send throat culture.
Monospot test or Epstein-Barr virus (EBV) titers to rule out infectious mononucleosis
Check LFT when EBV is the causative agent.

Neck x-ray: Anteroposterior/Lateral views to rule out soft tissue swelling, airway compromise, or obstruction.

- "Steeple sign" is seen when viral influenza causes croup.
- "Thumb sign" is seen when *H. influenzae* causes epiglottitis.

A Pharyngitis/Tonsillitis

Types:
- Viral pharyngitis/tonsillitis:
  - Most common causative agents include:
    - Adenoviruses
    - Epstein-Barr virus
    - Coxsackie virus
    - Herpes simplex virus
- Bacterial pharyngitis/tonsillitis:
  - Most common causative agents include:
    - Group A ß-hemolytic streptococci
    - Mycoplasma
    - *Haemophilus influenzae*
    - Chlamydia
    - Gonorrhea

P Start appropriate therapy based on the type of pharyngitis/tonsillitis identified

Recommend supportive care for viral infections:
- Pain relief with analgesics (acetaminophen, ibuprofen)
- Gargling with warm salt water or mouthwash can provide relief of symptoms.
- Lozenges or local anesthetic sprays can also be used for temporary relief.
- When EBV is detected, give additional recommendations:
  - Initiate oral steroids if airway compromise is suggested on exam.
  - Emphasize rest with no contact sports for one month.

Initiate antibiotic therapy along with supportive care for bacterial infections.
- Antibiotics used include:
  - Penicillin
  - Macrolides
  - Cephalosporins
- Administer intramuscular antibiotic, perform incision and drainage, or refer emergently to ENT.
  - Pts with a history of tonsillar abscess will usually require tonsillectomy in the future.

S   What complaints does the pt currently report?

Facial pain worsened with bending over, fever, chronic cough, halitosis, headache, purulent nasal discharge, or toothache can all be caused by sinusitis.

Symptoms of allergic rhinitis or recent upper respiratory infection lasting more than a week can be preludes to sinusitis.

Is the pt complaining of any dental problems?

Dental problems such as a tooth abscess, recent dental extractions, or dental work can lead to sinus infections.

Does the pt have nasal obstruction?

Inquire about a deviated nasal septum, nasal polyps, or large adenoids, which can all place the pt at risk for sinusitis.

Is the pt at risk for nosocomial infection?

Recent nasogastric or nasotracheal tube placement increases the pt's risk of acquiring sinusitis.

O   Check vital signs

Check for fever.

Perform physical exam

General: The pt may be mouth breathing because of nasal congestion.
HEENT:
- Palpate for tenderness of frontal or maxillary sinuses.
- There may be opacity of the affected sinus on transillumination.
- Nasal polyp or deviated nasal septum may be blocking the nasal passage.
- Swollen turbinates with purulent yellow or green discharge may be present.
- Oropharynx may have "cobblestoning" or visible streaks of mucopurulent discharge, indicating chronic postnasal drip.
- Inspect the eyes for periorbital swelling, erythema, and restriction of extraocular movements (orbital cellulitis).

Orbital cellulitis can be caused by direct spread of maxillary sinus infection, can lead to cavernous sinus thrombosis, and requires early recognition!

Consider the following labs and studies:

Sinus fluid culture obtained by sinus aspiration: aerobic, anaerobic, and fungal
X-ray of sinus series may reveal air-fluid levels, thickened mucosa, or sinus opacification.
CT scan of sinuses is reserved for pts who fail initial therapy, who are being considered for surgical intervention, or who have signs of periorbital/orbital cellulitis.

A **Sinusitis**
Types:
- Acute sinusitis
  - Sudden onset of symptoms listed above, especially after a recent upper respiratory infection
  - The most common bacteria involved:
    - *Streptococcus pneumoniae*
    - *Haemophilus influenzae*
    - *Moraxella catarrhalis*
    - Anaerobes
  - Suspect *Staphylococcus aureus* and gram-negative bacteria in nosocomial infection.
- Chronic sinusitis:
  - Symptoms persisting for three or more months
  - Besides the bacteria listed above, fungal species may be the cause.

P **Initiate pharmacotherapy**
Start antibiotics
- Amoxicillin
- Trimethoprim-sulfamethoxazole
- If no improvement on either therapy, prescribe:
  - Amoxicillin/clavulanic acid
  - Quinolones
  - Macrolides
Treatment duration
- Acute sinusitis will typically require 2 weeks.
- Chronic sinusitis will typically require 3 to 4 weeks.
Recommend ancillary therapies
- Intranasal steroids
- Oral decongestants
- Saline irrigation

Refer treatment failures to ears/nose/throat specialist
Endoscopic sinus surgery

S **What symptoms is the pt experiencing?**
Coughing, laughing, lifting, or sneezing can all be activities that precipitate the leakage of urine in stress incontinence.
Large amounts of urine are usually lost when the sensation of voiding is signaled in urge incontinence.
Dribbling after voiding or a feeling of incomplete voiding occurs with overflow incontinence.

Does the pt have signs suggesting a urinary tract infection (UTI)?
The presence of a UTI heralded by dysuria, frequency, urgency, and fever could be the cause of incontinence.

Review medical history
History of back injuries, cerebral vascular accidents, dementia, diabetes mellitus, and chronic UTIs can all contribute to urinary incontinence.

Has the pt undergone any surgeries?
Surgeries involving the back, pelvis, or urogenital tract lead to urinary incontinence.

Is the pt taking any medications that can cause cough, constipation, delirium, frequency, sedation, or urinary retention?
- Anticholingerics   - Antidepressants   - Antipsychotics
- Diuretics   - Hypnotics   - Opiates
- ACE inhibitors

How much alcohol or caffeinated beverages does the pt consume in 24 hours?
These two types of beverages are culprits of urinary incontinence because of their diuretic effect.

O **Perform physical exam**
Abdomen:
- Palpate for any masses or suprapubic tenderness.
- Distended bladder may be palpable when the urinary outflow tract is obstructed.
Pelvic:
- Atrophy of urethra or vaginal rugae may be seen in menopausal women.
- Assess pelvic floor muscle strength and check for cystocele, rectocele, or uterine prolapse.
- Check for the leakage of urine during a Valsalva maneuver.
Rectal:
- Perform digital rectal exam and check for enlarged prostate (benign prostatic hyperplasia), boggy or tender prostate (prostatitis), mass, or stool impaction.
- Assess sphincter tone: May be decreased in spinal cord injury.
Neuro:
- Examine lower extremity sensation, strength, and reflexes (anal wink).
- Perform Mini-Mental Status Exam to assess for possible dementia.

Consider the following labs and studies:
UA:
- Glucose suggests diabetes mellitus.
- Red blood cells suggest infection, stones, kidney trauma, or cancer.
- White blood cells suggest infection.

Urine culture to determine bacteria causing infection
Post-void residual: Introduce a catheter 10 minutes after voiding and measure the
residual volume obtained.
- Volume > 150 mL suggests hypotonic bladder or obstruction.

 Urinary Incontinence is involuntary loss of urine
Types:
- *Urge incontinence*: Caused by an overactive bladder, leading to intense urgency to void followed by a large amount of urine loss.
- *Stress incontinence*: Caused by inadequate internal urethral sphincter tone during increase of intra-abdominal pressure followed immediately by small amount of urine loss (e.g., coughing or sneezing).
- *Overflow incontinence*: Caused by distended bladder that may result from obstruction of urinary outflow tract or hypoactive bladder (e.g., benign prostatic hyperplasia [BPH], cystocele, urethral stricture, rectocele, mass, mass-effect of stool impaction, spinal cord injury, or neuropathy).
- Mixed: Involving a combination of the types above.

P Recommend behavioral modifications
Urinary diary: Used to record the number of times a pt voids, the frequency of accidents, the time and amount of fluid intake, and to schedule voids to establish control.
If pt has urge incontinence, start bladder retraining to suppress the urge by lengthening the interval between voids, increasing bladder capacity, and sitting down until the sensation passes.
Fluid modification and reduction of alcohol and caffeine consumption
Kegel exercises: repetitive maneuver of contracting the muscles of the rectum and vagina to recondition the pelvic floor muscles.

Start pharmacotherapy
Use anticholinergics for urge incontinence:
- Imipramine   - Oxybutynin
- Tolterodine   - Hyoscyamine
Use α-adrenergic agonists for stress incontinence:
- Pseudoephedrine   - Phenylpropanolamine
Use α-adrenergic antagonists for overflow incontinence caused by BPH:
- Doxazosin   - Terazosin

Refer depending on the cause of incontinence
Gynecologist: Fit a pessary in uterine prolapse.
Urologist: Perform transurethral resection of the prostate in a pt with severe BPH.
Neurosurgeon: Perform discectomy to relieve spinal cord compression.

S **Does the pt present with symptoms of a urinary tract infection (UTI)?**
Common symptoms of frequency, urgency, and dysuria can be present in a UTI.
Other possible associated symptoms include fever, nausea, vomiting, hematuria,
  urinary incontinence, and foul-smelling urine.

If there is pain, where is it located?
Lower abdominal or suprapubic areas can indicate cystitis.
Low-back pain or flank pain can suggest pyelonephritis.
Urethral pain can be present in urethritis.

Has the pt had many UTIs?
Recurrent UTIs may indicate urologic abnormalities, such as ureteral reflux, stag-horn
  calculus, struvite, or fistula.

Is the pt sexually active?
In pts with complaints of vaginal or penile discharge, a sexually transmitted infection
  (STI) can be responsible for a UTI.
Contraceptive use of barrier methods such as condoms or diaphragms with
  spermicides can cause local irritation, which may lead to dysuria.
Some pts can have an allergic reaction to latex condoms.

Any possibility of pregnancy?
Pregnancy makes women prone to UTIs because of the dilating effects of progesterone
  on the smooth muscle.

Has the pt had any recent trauma to the urogenital tract?
Pts with recent instrumentation or catheterization are susceptible to UTIs.

Inquire about the presence of air with urination (pneumaturia)
Fistulas can develop between the bladder and nearby anatomic structures.

Is there a history of abdominal or pelvic surgeries?
There can be increased risks for UTIs after surgical manipulations of bladder, uterus,
  kidney, or pelvic structures.

O **Perform physical exam**
Abdomen: Check for surgical scars and suprapubic tenderness.
Back: Palpate costovertebral angle tenderness (CVAT).
GU:
  - If female, search for any urethral lesions or vaginal discharge.
  - If male, search for lesions on the penis or urethral meatus.
  - Palpate each epididymis for tenderness (epididymitis).
Rectal:
  - If male, palpate the prostate for tenderness (prostatitis).
  - See Epididymitis/Prostatitis (p. 30) for specifics.

Consider the following labs and studies:
UA suggestive of infection:
- Bacteria	- Nitrite positive
- Blood	- Leukocyte esterase positive

Send urine culture if initial urine dip suggests infection.
Collect gonorrhea/chlamydia cultures if history or physical exam indicates risk.
If the pt has a history of multiple UTIs, CVAT, or nephrolithiasis, consider renal
  ultrasound or IV pyelogram.

A **Urinary Tract Infection**
Types
- Lower UTI: Infection restricted to the bladder (cystitis)
  - Typical symptoms include dysuria, frequency, or urgency.
- Upper UTI: Infection involving the kidney (pyelonephritis)
  - Typical symptoms include the ones listed above along with fever, flank pain, and low-back pain.
- Most UTIs are caused by gram-negative bacteria:
  - *Escherichia coli*
  - *Klebsiella*
  - *Proteus*
- Most common gram-positive bacteria involved are:
  - *Enterococci*
  - *Staphylococcus aureus*
  - *Staphylococcus saprophyticus*

P **Start a 3- to 7-day course of antibiotics when a lower UTI is identified (see STI p. 94)**

- Trimethoprim-sulfamethoxazole	- Cephalosporin
- Quinolone	- Nitrofurantoin

Treat uncomplicated upper UTIs with a 10- to 14-day course of antibiotics
Admit severely ill-appearing pts for IV antibiotics until pt is afebrile for 24 hours.
- Oral medications can then be continued for a total of 14 days.

Treat both the pt and the partner with appropriate antibiotics if an STI is identified.
Gonorrhea: Ceftriaxone or quinolone
Chlamydia: Doxycycline, macrolide, or quinolone

A one-time dose of 2 g azithromycin can be used to treat both infections, but increased GI side effects may ensue.

Tailor antibiotics to urine-culture sensitivities once available.

II

Obstetrics & Gynecology

S **Obtain identifying data**
Age, female, occupation, and marital status

Obtain full history
HPI: Obtain a complete history of the pt's illness.
- Refer to specific topics for guidance.

PMH: List any medical problems and hospitalizations.
PSH: Has the pt had any surgeries or minor procedures?
Allergies: Any known drug allergies?
Medications:
- Is the pt currently taking any drugs, prescribed, or over-the-counter?
- Is the pt taking any herbals, supplements, or vitamins?

FH: Is there a history of breast cancer, colon cancer, diabetes mellitus, heart disease, hypertension, hyperlipidemia, or osteoporosis?
SH:
- Does the pt use alcohol, tobacco, or drugs?
  - If yes, quantify the amounts, the frequency, and for how long.
- What is the pt's marital status?
- What is the pt's occupation?

Ob/Gyn:
- Age of menarche?
- Frequency, duration, and blood flow of menstrual period?
- Age of first pregnancy?
- Age of first sexual encounter?
- Number of lifetime sexual partners?
- Gender of partners: Male, female, or both?
- Number of pregnancies, deliveries, abortions?
- History of sexually transmitted infections?
- Methods of contraceptives used in the past and in the present (if sexually active)?
- When was the pt's most recent Papanicolaou test?
  - Normal results?

GHM:
- Has the pt ever had a mammogram?
  - If yes, was it normal?
- Review the pt's immunization record and last tuberculosis test.
- Has the pt had fecal occult blood testing (FOBT), colonoscopy, or bone mineral density measurement if age appropriate?

ROS: Review each organ system (See Adult History & Physical p. 2)

O **Check vital signs**
Height, weight, body mass index

Perform physical exam
Full physical to include clinical breast exam and pelvic exam when indicated

Consider the following labs and studies:

- CBC for anemia	- Chemistry panel for electrolyte abnormalities
- Lipid panel	- Liver panel
- Papanicolaou test	- TSH if thyroid disease suspected
- Rapid plasma reagin	- FOBT if over 50 years old
- ECG	- CXR

A Well woman exam

P Implement preventive measures

Breast cancer screen
- Breast self-exam: Monthly
- Mammogram: Starting at age 40 every 1 to 2 years

Cervical cancer screen
- Papanicolaou test: Every 1 to 3 years depending on risk
  - May need to be done more frequently if abnormality detected
  - Begin at the age when pt becomes sexually active or at age 21 (whichever comes first).
  - Can discontinue at age 65 if tests have been consistently normal in the previous 10 years.

Osteoporosis
- Bone mineral density measurement
  - Starting at age 65
  - Start younger if pt has risk factors:
    - Previous spinal fracture, family history, low body weight, smoker

Colorectal cancer screen, immunizations, dental care, vision care, and hearing care (See Adult History & Physical p. 2)

Start behavioral and dietary modifications:

Calcium supplementation
Diet and exercise
Smoking cessation
Skin protection
Folic acid supplementation if pt is of childbearing age and able to become pregnant
Family planning if pt is of childbearing age

S   Obtain a detailed history during initial visit

HPI:

- Is this a desired pregnancy?
- When was the pt's last normal menstrual period?
  - ◆ Is she sure about her dates?
  - ◆ Was she using contraception?
- Inquire about any current symptoms associated with pregnancy
  - ◆ Nausea, vomiting, constipation, breast tenderness, or fatigue?
- Ask about any complications
  - ◆ Any abdominal pain, cramping, vaginal bleeding, or discharge?

PMH: Any history of:

- Asthma	- Diabetes mellitus
- Hypertension	- Heart disease
- Kidney disease	- Seizure disorder
- Thyroid disease	

PSH: Any abdominal or pelvic surgeries?

Allergies: Any known drug allergies?

Medications: Is the pt taking any prescribed or over-the-counter medications?

FMH: Inquire about any inheritable genetic disorders in the expectant mother's family
and the expectant father's family:

- Cystic fibrosis	- Down syndrome
- Hemophilia	- Muscular dystrophy
- Sickle cell disease or trait	- Tay-Sachs

SH:

- What is the pt's ethnic background?
- Is the pt married? Does she know who the father is? Does the father know?
- Is the pt working? Any exposure to harmful fumes or chemicals?
- Any use of alcohol, drugs, or tobacco? (Quantify)
- Are there pets at home?

Ob/Gyn history: Obtain a complete history of prior pregnancies.

- Total number of pregnancies: Delivered, aborted, or miscarried?
- Normal spontaneous vaginal delivery or cesarean section?
  - ◆ Length of labor?
  - ◆ Gestational age, birth weight, and height?
  - ◆ Any anesthesia used?
  - ◆ Any complications?
- Ectopic pregnancy or multiple births?
- Any history of abnormal Papanicolaou test or sexually transmitted infections?
- How many sexual partners?

ROS: Review each organ system.

O   Check vital signs

Check for hypertension and fever.

Weight (compare to prepregnancy weight)

Perform complete physical exam (focus on areas listed below)

HEENT: Palpate for thyromegaly.

Chest: Auscultate for wheezing or crackles.

Heart: Listen for a murmur or abnormal heart sounds.

Abdomen: Palpate fundus of uterus and measure fundal height.
  • Attempt to detect fetal heart tones by Doppler.
Pelvic: Examine for external lesions or discharge and perform bimanual exam for cervical motion tenderness, adnexal mass, and uterine size.
Pelvic type: Determine if gynecoid, anthropoid, android, or platypelloid shape.
Extremities: Observe for edema.

Consider the following labs and studies:
  • 1st trimester labs to be obtained at initial visit:

- Blood type, Rh, antibody screen	- Rubella titer
- CBC	- HIV
- Hepatitis B titers	- Gonorrhea and chlamydia cultures
- Papanicolaou test	- 1-hour glucose test if at risk
- UA with culture	

  - Venereal disease research laboratory/rapid plasma reagin
  - Pelvic ultrasound if unsure of pregnancy dates or if there is size discrepancy

A **1st Trimester Visit: Intrauterine Pregnancy at ___ weeks (1 to 12 weeks)**
Document if advanced maternal age (≥ 35 years), teenage pregnancy, or late in starting prenatal care.

P **At the initial visit, the gestational age of the fetus is estimated by comparing the size of the uterus to the date of the last menstrual period.**

Subsequent 1st trimester prenatal care visits will require checking:
- Cumulative weight gain	- Blood pressure check
- Urine dipstick test	- Fetal heart tones and fundal height

Offer genetics counseling to women with:
- Advanced maternal age	- Family history of genetic/inherited disorders
- Exposure to teratogens	- Personal history of genetic/inherited disorders

  - These women may be offered chorionic villus sampling or amniocentesis

Discuss the risk of 1st trimester bleeding (See Bleeding during Pregnancy p. 74)
Counsel regarding:
- Bathing	- Drug use	- Toxoplasmosis in cat feces
- Exercise	- Nutrition	- Prenatal vitamin use
- Morning sickness	- Travel	
- Sexual intercourse	- Over-the-counter medications	

Place tuberculosis skin test
If positive, defer CXR until second trimester.

Return to clinic in 4 weeks or sooner if any complications develop

S **Are symptoms from the 1st trimester improving?**
Common symptoms in the 1st trimester are nausea, vomiting, constipation, breast tenderness, and fatigue.

Does the pt complain of abdominal pain, vaginal bleeding, or loss of fluid?
These symptoms may indicate threatened abortion.

Any vaginal discharge, fever, pelvic pressure, urinary symptoms, or back pain?
Pregnancy can increase pt's risk for urinary tract infections.

Is there fetal movement?
Usually perceived around 16 weeks

Does the pt have new complaints or concerns?
Round ligament pain:
- Pain secondary to the rapid growth of the uterus, resulting in stretching of the round ligament

Gastroesophageal reflux disease (GERD):
- Pain caused by regurgitation of stomach acid into the esophagus because of increased intra-abdominal pressure and lower esophageal relaxation

O **Check vital signs**
Check for hypertension, fever, or tachycardia.
Calculate total weight gained (compare to prepregnancy weight).

Perform physical exam
Chest: Auscultate for wheezing or crackles.
Heart: Listen for a murmur or abnormal heart sounds.
Abdomen:
- Palpate and measure fundus of uterus.
- Document if fetal heart tones are detected by Doppler.

Pelvic:
- Inspect if history of vaginal bleeding, contractions, or discharge.
- Examine for discharge, blood, and cervical motion tenderness.
- Check for open or closed os.

Extremities: Observe for edema.

Consider the following labs and studies:
CBC for anemia
1-hr glucose test to rule out gestational diabetes (usually presents > 20 weeks)
Maternal serum α-fetoprotein/quadruple screen at 15 to 20 weeks
If PPD is positive, obtain CXR with abdominal shield after 20 weeks.

If Rh negative, recheck antibody screen at 26 to 28 weeks.
- If still negative, can administer RhoGAM at 28 weeks.

A **2nd Trimester Visit, Intrauterine pregnancy at ___weeks (13 to 28 weeks)**
Document problems in second trimester such as:
Rh-negative status
Abnormal quadruple screen
Round ligament pain
GERD
Low-back pain

P **2nd trimester prenatal care visits will require checking:**
Cumulative weight gain
Blood pressure check
Urine dipstick test
Fetal heart tones and fundal height

Offer genetics counseling to women who have:
Advanced maternal age
Family history of genetic/inherited disorder
Exposure to teratogens
Personal history of genetic/inherited disorder
Missed quadruple screen
These women are offered chorionic villus sampling or amniocentesis.

Counsel regarding:

- Bathing	- Drug use
- Toxoplasmosis in cat feces	- Exercise
- Nutrition	- Prenatal vitamin use
- Morning sickness	- Travel
- Sexual intercourse	- Over-the-counter medications

If pt has large increase in weight or no increase in weight, refer to nutritionist
Underweight pt should gain about 30 to 40 pounds.
Normal-weight pt should gain about 25 to 35 pounds.
Overweight pt should gain about 15 to 25 pounds.
Obese pt should gain no more than 15 pounds.

Treat specific problems:

Administer RhoGAM if Rh negative and antibody screen negative.

Use acetaminophen for round ligament pain.
Encourage smaller, frequent meals, upright posture for 2 to 3 hours after a meal, and use of antacids for GERD.
Start back exercises, use prescribed girdle, and use acetaminophen for low-back pain.

Return to clinic in 4 weeks or sooner if any complications develop

S **Does the pt have any symptoms that may indicate labor or complications?**

Complications include:

- Abdominal pain	- Cramping	- Vaginal bleeding
- Discharge	- Fever	- Pelvic pressure
- Urinary symptoms	- Low-back pain	- Leakage of fluid

Any fetal movement?
Baby should kick 10 times in 2 hours.

Does the pt have new complaints or concerns?

Braxton Hicks contractions

- Spontaneous tightening of uterine muscles anywhere from 30 to 60 seconds
- These contractions are thought to play a part in toning the uterine muscle and promoting the flow of blood to the placenta.
- Sometimes called "false labor" or "practice contractions"

O **Check vital signs**
Check for hypertension and fever.
Calculate total weight gained (compare to prepregnancy weight).

Perform physical exam
Chest: Auscultate for wheezing or crackles.
Heart: Listen for a murmur or abnormal heart sounds.
Abdomen: Palpate and measure fundus of uterus.
- Document fetal heart tones and Leopold's.
Pelvic:
- Inspect only if pt reports any vaginal bleeding, contractions, discharge, leakage of fluid, or if unable to tell by Leopold maneuvers the position of the baby.
- Palpate for an open os or cervical motion tenderness.
- Check station, effacement, and dilation.
- Perform sterile speculum exam to check for discharge, blood, and pooling.
Extremities: Check for edema.

Consider the following labs and studies:
CBC for anemia
Repeat gonorrhea, chlamydia, and VDRL in high-risk pt
Collect group B streptococcus culture ($\geq$ 35 weeks)

A 3rd Trimester Visit: Intrauterine pregnancy at ___weeks (29 to 40 weeks)
Document problems in 2nd trimester such as:
Rupture of membranes
Vertex or breech presentation
Group B Streptococcus (GBS)–positive mother

P **3rd trimester prenatal care visits will require checking:**
Cumulative weight gain
Blood pressure check
Urine dipstick test
Leopold maneuvers
Fetal heart tones and fundal height

Treat specific problems
If pt reports leakage of fluid, need to rule out rupture of membranes:
- Perform sterile speculum exam and check for:
  - Pooling in vaginal vault
  - Nitrazine paper test
  - Ferning on a slide
If baby is not in vertex position:
- Wait and see if baby changes position before delivery.
- Refer for external version.
- Schedule cesarean section.
If mother is GBS positive:
- Will need to give intravenous antibiotic prophylaxis antepartum.

Counsel regarding:
- Bathing	- Drug use
- Toxoplasmosis in cat feces	- Exercise
- Nutrition	- Prenatal vitamin use
- Morning sickness	- Travel
- Sexual intercourse	- Over-the-counter medications
- Birth plan	- Preterm labor and labor precautions

- Encourage fluids or change in activity when feeling Braxton Hicks contractions.

Return to clinic every 2 to 3 weeks between 29 to 35 weeks and then every week until the delivery date
If the pt begins to have contractions, leakage of fluid, vaginal bleeding, or decreased fetal movement, report to ER

S **Obtain a detailed menstrual history**
It is important to gather information regarding the pt's frequency, duration, and last menstrual period, if pt has had menarche.
Menopause can present with vaginal dryness, hot flashes, and missed periods.

Is the pt sexually active?

A common cause of amenorrhea can be pregnancy.

It is important to obtain information about prior pregnancy or infertility.

Has the pt undergone uterine instrumentation?
After dilation and curettage, pts may develop *Asherman syndrome*.

Are there symptoms of severe headaches, visual disturbances, or galactorrhea?
These symptoms can suggest a pituitary adenoma.

Any recent weight change?
Women with drastic weight change caused by dieting or participation in competitive sports are susceptible to irregular periods.
Eating disorders such as bulimia and anorexia can cause amenorrhea.

Did the pt ever have an illness requiring chemotherapy or radiation?
These treatments may cause gonadal failure.

Does the pt complain of associated hair loss, weight gain, cold intolerance, or constipation?
These symptoms may be evident in hypothyroidism.

Review medications
Women using hormones, illicit drugs, or diet pills can have interruptions in their menstrual cycles.

O **Perform physical exam**
General: Check pt's habitus.
HEENT:
- Erosion of teeth may indicate chronic vomiting.
- Visual fields may be disturbed if pituitary is enlarged.
- Check thyroid for masses or goiter.
- Short, webbed neck is consistent with *Turner syndrome*.

Chest:
- Quantify Tanner stage.
- Express nipples for galactorrhea if suspected prolactinoma.

Abdomen: Palpate for masses.
Pelvic:
- Quantify Tanner stage.
- Inspect external and internal genitalia to ensure normal outflow tract.
- Palpate uterus and adnexa to rule out masses.

Skin:
- Inspect for hirsutism or acne, suggesting polycystic ovarian syndrome (PCOS).
- Brittle hair, nails, or dry skin may indicate hypothyroidism.
- Repetitive self-induced vomiting may cause calluses on the dorsum of fingers.

Consider the following labs and studies:
Urine pregnancy test
Prolactin is elevated when there is a prolactinoma.
Follicle-stimulating hormone (FSH) is elevated in ovarian failure (FSH > 40).
Luteinizing hormone (LH) is elevated in PCOS (LH > 35).
Thyroid-stimulating hormone (TSH) is elevated in hypothyroidism.

 Amenorrhea
Primary amenorrhea: The absence of menarche (menarche usually occurs by 16 years
  of age). Possible etiologies include:
       - Imperforate hymen   - *Turner syndrome*
       - Testicular feminization   - Transvaginal septum
Secondary amenorrhea: The absence of menses for at least 3 months in a pt who has
  menstruated before
Limited differential diagnosis of an extensive list includes:
       - *Cushing's syndrome*   - Hypothyroidism
       - Eating disorder (anorexia or bulimia)   - Excessive exercise
       - Obesity   - PCOS
       - Pregnancy   - Prolactinoma
       - Stress   - *Turner syndrome*
       - *Asherman syndrome*   - Premature ovarian failure
       - Menopause

 Determine if the pt has primary or secondary amenorrhea
Rule out pregnancy.

Use laboratory test and studies to determine the cause of amenorrhea
See laboratory studies listed above.

Perform progesterone challenge test in secondary amenorrhea
If withdrawal bleeding occurs in less than 2 weeks, the test is positive, indicating that
  the pt has adequate estrogen and is having anovulation.
Give the pt oral contraceptives or low-dose hormones to regulate the cycles.

Treat by addressing the underlying cause
Recommend calcium supplementation

S **How far along is the pregnancy during the episode of bleeding?**
Identifying the trimester during which the bleeding occurred may assist in delineating
   the cause.
Bleeding may be accompanied by contractions, cramps, pain, or pelvic pressure.
Pt can have various amounts of bleeding, ranging from spotting to hemorrhaging.

Did the bleeding occur after a specific event?
Recent trauma such as automobile accidents, falls, or intercourse can precipitate
   bleeding.

Abruption of the placenta can present with painful bleeding.

Has the pt had abnormal or malodorous vaginal discharge?
Sexually transmitted infection (STIs) can cause ectopic pregnancy or cervicitis, which
   can lead to bleeding.

**Has the pt had other episodes of bleeding throughout this pregnancy
or in prior pregnancies?**
Pts with placenta previa are at risk for bleeding throughout the pregnancy.
History of cesarean section or multigravida places the pt at risk for uterine rupture in
   the last trimester.

Obtain social history
Has the pt been using alcohol, tobacco, or drugs?

O **Check vital signs**
Check if the pt is hemodynamically stable.

Perform physical exam
General: Pt may be pale or toxic appearing.
Heart: Tachycardia and flow murmurs can be present in high-output states.
Abdomen:
   • Examine for tenderness.
   • Search for doptones and palpate the uterine fundus.
Pelvic:
   • Determine the site of bleeding.
   • Inspect if the cervical os is open, which can indicate spontaneous abortion.
   • Palpate the adnexa for masses, which can suggest ectopic pregnancy.
   • Check for abnormal discharge.
   • Perform a sterile speculum exam to check for pooling, ferning, and nitrazine
     tests if placenta previa not suspected.

Consider the following labs and studies:
CBC to determine if anemia or infection is present
Quantitative β-hCG for baseline level
Gonorrhea and chlamydia cultures if discharge is present
Transabdominal/pelvic ultrasound

Bleeding during pregnancy
1st trimester bleeding's differential diagnosis
Cervicitis: STIs can cause inflammation and bleeding of the cervix.
Ectopic pregnancy: Implantation of the fertilized egg outside the uterine cavity
   presenting with unilateral pelvic pain and bleeding
Molar pregnancy: Gestational trophoblastic tissue, which can have abnormal fetal
   tissue, malignant invasive potential, and heavy or irregular bleeding
Postcoital bleeding: Bleeding that happens after intercourse caused by a friable cervix
Spontaneous abortion: Loss of intrauterine pregnancy, which presents with bleeding
Threatened abortion: Term used to describe bleeding before 20 weeks' gestation that
   presents with closed cervical os without loss of fetus

3rd trimester bleeding's differential diagnosis
Bloody show: Spotting or bleeding that presents with contractions at the onset of labor
Abruptio placentae: Placental separation from the uterine wall, resulting in *painful*
   bleeding usually in the 3rd trimester
Placenta previa: Placenta that develops over the cervical os and results in *painless*
   bleeding
Uterine rupture: Presents with intense abdominal and pelvic pain and may have
   associated vaginal spotting, bleeding, or hemorrhage
Note: 2nd trimester bleeding may be a result of any cause listed above.

P **The management of bleeding during pregnancy depends on which**
trimester the pt is in and the severity of the bleeding
1st trimester bleeding
Ensure that this is not a molar pregnancy or an ectopic pregnancy.
Serial β-hCG levels are checked in 48 hours to ensure that the level is rising.
   • Doubles every 48 hours early in the pregnancy
   • Failure to increase by 66% means pregnancy is not progressing normally.
Pelvic rest is recommended.
RhoGAM is administered if pt is Rh negative.

Spontaneous abortion (1st or 2nd trimester)
Pt can wait for the products of conception to be expelled if early on.
Pt can be referred to Ob/Gyn specialist for intervention.

3rd trimester bleeding
All will require evaluation in labor and delivery.
The pt will be monitored for contractions.
The fetus will be evaluated on the fetal heart monitor for distress.
The pt may require immediate surgical intervention.

S **When did the symptoms begin?**
Dysfunctional uterine bleeding (DUB) is common around the time of menarche and menopause.
Have the pt quantify amount of bleeding (tampons or pads used in 24 hours).

Is the pt sexually active?
An ectopic pregnancy can present with abnormal uterine bleeding.
Women who have undergone a recent abortion can have DUB.

Does the pt have any preexisting medical problems?
Thyroid disease, adrenal disease, liver disease, blood dyscrasia, and prolactinoma can all be primary causes of uterine bleeding.

What medications is the pt using?
Medroxyprogesterone injections can give pts erratic uterine bleeding.
The use of anticoagulants such as coumadin or heparin can lead to abnormal uterine bleeding when the levels of prothrombin time (PT) and partial thromboplastin time (PTT) are elevated.

Has the pt had any devices or foreign bodies inserted into the vagina?
Bleeding can be a result of trauma to the tissues inside of the vagina.
An intrauterine device (IUD) can potentially be a cause of abnormal uterine bleeding.

O **Check vital signs**
Ensure that the pt is hemodynamically stable.

Perform physical exam
General: Pt may look pale, toxic appearing, or obese.
HEENT:
  • Check visual fields (abnormality can indicate pituitary adenoma).
  • Palpate the thyroid for enlargement or nodules.
Heart: Tachycardia or flow murmur may be present in high-output states.
Abdomen: Palpate for masses.
Pelvic:
  • Inspect the external skin and internal vaginal walls for bruising, lesions, lacerations, or foreign bodies.
  • Identify if blood is flowing from the cervical os and check for cervical motion tenderness.
  • Determine if the uterus is enlarged or globular, suggesting fibroids.
  • Palpate adnexa for masses or tenderness.
Skin: Survey for ecchymosis (blood dyscrasia or abuse).

Consider the following labs and studies:
CBC to determine presence of anemia.
Urine pregnancy test must be done to rule out pregnancy.
LFT/PT/PTT to rule out liver disease and coagulopathy
FSH if menopause is suspected
TSH to rule out thyroid disease
Prolactin to rule out prolactinoma
Pelvic ultrasound if indicated by findings on physical exam

Dysfunctional Uterine Bleeding

This term is used to describe abnormal uterine bleeding when no other cause or uterine abnormality is found.

Specific terms used to describe DUB:
- *Menorrhagia*: Heavier bleeding during a normal cycle
- *Metrorrhagia*: Frequent bleeding or spotting before expected cycles
- *Oligomenorrhea*: Bleeding that occurs after a 35-day interval
- *Polymenorrhea*: Bleeding that occurs before a 21-day interval

Usually occurs around the time of menarche and menopause during anovulation

Diagnosis of exclusion when differential diagnosis is exhausted:
- No chronic or constitutional disease: Kidney, liver disease, or eating disorder
- No endocrine disease: Prolactinoma or thyroid disease
- No medications: Contraceptive hormones, coumadin, or heparin
- No pregnancy: Intrauterine, ectopic, or molar
- No foreign bodies or trauma: Intrauterine device or laceration
- No tumors: Uterine cancer, fibroids, or polyps

P **Treat as an outpatient if vital signs are stable and no hemorrhaging is present**

If there is history of long-term anovulation or the pt is older than 35 years, endometrial biopsy is necessary to rule out endometrial hyperplasia or carcinoma.

Start hormones and NSAIDs to control the bleeding:
Estrogen therapy:
- In the acute setting, use conjugated estrogen 35 μg or higher every 8 hours for one week.
- Once bleeding stops, use hormone replacement therapy in women age 50 or older if there are no contraindications.

Progesterone therapy:
- In the acute setting, use medroxyprogesterone acetate (Provera) 10 mg po daily the week following estrogen therapy.
- Continue with combination contraceptive pills for at least three cycles.
- If estrogen is not tolerated or contraindicated, can cycle the pt with Provera 10 mg daily for 10 days at least every 4 months.

Other therapies include
Progestin IUD

Antigonadotropin therapy with Danocrine

Admit pt to hospital if bleeding is severe or endometrial cancer is suspected
Interventions may include dilation and curettage, endometrial ablation, or hysterectomy.

S **When did the dysmenorrhea or pelvic pain begin?**

After menarche, primary dysmenorrhea is accompanied by symptoms such as headache, nausea, vomiting, diarrhea, breast tenderness, and pain in the lower back or legs.

These symptoms coincide with the start of ovulatory cycles, usually beginning within 6 to 12 months after menarche.

Are the symptoms related to the pt's menstrual cycle?

Symptoms of primary dysmenorrhea usually occur during the first days of menses.

Is the pt sexually active?

Abnormal vaginal discharge, a history of multiple sexual partners, and pelvic pain can suggest a sexually transmitted infection (STI) or pelvic inflammatory disease (PID).

What type of contraceptive method does the pt use?

An intrauterine device (IUD) can be a cause of pelvic pain.

Has the pt had any abdominal or pelvic surgeries?

Adhesions can cause pelvic pain.

Has the pt ever been pregnant?

Primary dysmenorrhea can disappear after first childbirth and may mitigate with increasing age.

Pelvic pain with intercourse (dyspareunia) and infertility can point to endometriosis.

Does the pt have any systemic symptoms?

When pelvic pain is present, GI, GU, and Gyn etiologies must be investigated.

O **Perorm physical exam**

Abdomen: Palpate for peritoneal signs or masses.

Pelvic:

- Check for abnormal discharge, cervical motion tenderness (*chandelier sign*) which points to PID.
- Adnexal enlargement or tenderness may indicate ectopic pregnancy, salpingitis, or tubo-ovarian abscess.
- Palpable uterine enlargement, firm mass, or globular shape can suggest uterine fibroids.
- Probe the cervical os if it appears stenotic.

Rectal: Perform a digital rectal exam to check for masses, tenderness, or positive guaiac.

Consider the following labs and studies:

CBC to rule out infection

UA and urine pregnancy test

Gonorrhea and chlamydia cultures

Pelvic ultrasound if there are any structural abnormalities on the physical exam

A **Dysmenorrhea**

Primary Dysmenorrhea

- Cyclic uterine pain that usually begins around the time of menarche
- Described as cramping pain occurring around the time of menstruation for about 2 to 3 days
- Pt has a normal pelvic exam and no organic disease is identified.
- Caused by prostaglandins typed as $PGF_{2\alpha}$

  ♦ Stimulates uterine contraction and tonicity
  ♦ Leads to uterine ischemia and an increase in nerve ending sensitivity
Secondary Dysmenorrhea
  • Uterine pain beginning years after menarche as a result of organic disease
  • May have abnormality on pelvic examination
  • Causes:
    ♦ Adenomyosis
    ♦ Cervical stenosis
    ♦ Ectopic pregnancy
    ♦ Endometriosis
    ♦ Fibroids/polyps
    ♦ IUD
    ♦ PID
    ♦ Tubo-ovarian abscess
    ♦ Salpingitis
Pelvic Pain
  • Acute: Pain that develops within hours to days in lower abdominal quadrants
    ♦ Causes:
      - Appendicitis   - Diverticular disease   - Ectopic pregnancy
      - PID   - Tubo-ovarian abscess   - Intestinal obstruction
      - Nephrolithiasis   - Ruptured ovarian cyst   - Spontaneous abortion
      - Urinary tract infection
  • Chronic: Recurrent pain present at least 6 months in lower abdominal quadrants
    ♦ Causes:
      - Adenomyosis   - Irritable bowel syndrome   - Adhesions
      - Fibroids   - Primary dysmenorrhea   - Interstitial cystitis
      - Endometriosis   - Inflammatory bowel disease

P **Start pharmacotherapy to treat primary dysmenorrhea**
NSAIDs and COX-2 inhibitors
  • Work by inhibiting prostaglandin production
Contraceptives
  • Oral contraceptive pills: Effective symptom reduction in 90% of pts
  • Progesterone-containing IUD: Assess if pt is at risk for STIs before insertion.
Nutritional supplements: Vitamin E and omega-3 fatty acids
Complimentary/alternative medicine: Acupuncture

Treat the underlying cause in secondary dysmenorrhea or other pelvic pains
Surgical intervention:
  • Necessary for secondary dysmenorrhea and acute or chronic pelvic pain
    requiring procedural attention, for example:
    ♦ Cervical stenosis: Dilation
    ♦ Ovarian cyst: Cystectomy
    ♦ Fibroids: Fibroidectomy/hysterectomy

S **Has the pt used any method of contraception in the past?**
Pts may mention reasons for discontinuation, side effects, inconveniences, breakthrough bleeding, and efficacy of prior methods.

Does the pt have a particular method in mind?
Pt preference may increase adherence.

This may be an optimal time to dispel myths about contraception.

Does the pt have a significant past medical history?
Pts who have a history of breast cancer, endometrial cancer, hypertension, hyperlipidemia, liver disease, stroke, venous thrombosis, or migraine headaches must consider the risks and benefits of hormones versus other methods.

Obtain Ob/Gyn history
See Well Woman Exam (p. 64).
Determine if all pregnancies have been planned.

Obtain social history
The use of tobacco and hormones is contraindicated in women ≥ 35 years.

O **Check vital signs**
Check if pt is hypertensive.

Perform physical exam
Perform breast and pelvic exams (see Well Woman Exam p. 64).

Consider the following labs and studies:
- CBC
- Papanicolaou test
- Gonorrhea and chlamydia cultures
- Lipid panel
- Urine pregnancy test
- Mammogram (pt ≥ 40 years)
- Offer hepatitis B and C, HIV, and syphilis testing if pt is at high risk
  for sexually transmitted infection (STIs).

A **Family Planning**
Use of a contraceptive method to prevent unwanted pregnancy

P **Consider the following factors before choosing a form of contraception**
Desire or preference
Past experiences and failures
Lifestyle
Cultural beliefs
Religious beliefs
Cost

None of the contraceptive methods listed below are 100% effective except for abstinence, and all of the methods have advantages and disadvantages
Abstinence: No intercourse
Barrier methods: Methods that prevent pregnancy by blocking the sperm from entering the uterus and fertilizing the oocyte.
- *Condoms*: Preferred method for new or nonmonogamous partners
  - Used with a spermicide
  - Need to be applied before penetration and removed before detumescence
  - Prevents STIs

- *Diaphragm*: Used with a spermicide
  - ✦ Placed < 6 hours before intercourse
  - ✦ Can be used for 24 hours
- *Cervical cap*: Used with a spermicide
  - ✦ Placed < 6 hours before intercourse
  - ✦ Can be used for 48 hours

Coitus interruptus: Withdrawal of the penis before ejaculation occurs

Hormones: Female hormones that are formulated with estrogen and progesterone in combination or progesterone alone to prevent ovulation from occurring

- Available in the form of pills, patches, cervical rings, or injections
- *Emergency contraception*: Higher hormone doses that are used 12 hours apart to inhibit or delay ovulation, prevent the sperm from fertilizing the oocyte, or impair implantation.
  - ✦ Must be taken within 72 hours of unprotected intercourse

Intrauterine device: A device that is inserted into the pt's uterus

- Not recommended for pts with an STI or at high risk for exposure
- Unclear mechanism of action that seems to prevent fertilization

Natural family planning (also referred to as the "rhythm method"): Relies on the female partner having regular cycles and abstaining during the fertilization window

- Basal body temperature
- Cervical mucus

Sterilization: A permanent form of contraception that requires that the fallopian tubes be ligated, clipped, or cut to prevent the oocyte from reaching the uterus

Instruct pt

Discuss the risks and benefits of each method.

Inform the pt how to use each method effectively.

Educate the pt on STI prevention.

S **How long has the couple been trying to conceive?**
More than 80% of couples will conceive within 12 months.

What past medical histories do each of the partners have?
Women who have had sexually transmitted infections are at a higher risk of tubal
  scarring.
Men who experienced mumps orchitis in pubertal or adult life undergo damage to the
  reproductive function of the testis.
Endocrine disorders of the adrenals, pituitary, or thyroid can cause infertility.
  • Eating disorders disrupt the hypothalamic-pituitary-gonadal axis.
Exposure to chemicals, radiation, or extreme temperatures can affect fertility.

Has either partner undergone surgical procedures?
Abdominal or pelvic surgeries involving ectopic pregnancy, fibroids, ovarian cysts,
  dilation and curettage, hernia repair, tubal ligation reversal, or vasectomy reversal can
  all contribute to infertility.

Does the woman have regular menstrual cycles?
Women who have anovulatory states may have irregular cycles.
Pts who used medroxyprogesterone injections may have abnormal ovulatory cycles
  that may take up to 18 months to normalize.

 Perform physical exam
HEENT:
  • Test for visual field defects that can indicate pituitary adenoma.
  • Palpate for thyroid masses or nodules.
Breast: Check for galactorrhea.
Pelvic:
  • Inspect vaginal vault for mucopurulent discharge.
  • Ensure that uterus and adnexa are not enlarged and that cervix is patent.
Urogenital:
  • Inspect the male urethral meatus for mucopurulent discharge.
  • Document the size of each testicle, and check for varicoceles.
  • Palpate each epididymis and the prostate for tenderness.

Consider the following labs and studies:
Gonorrhea and chlamydia cultures
TSH and prolactin levels to rule out thyroid and pituitary involvement
Pelvic ultrasound if female exam indicates a structural abnormality

A **Infertility is the inability to conceive after one year of unprotected intercourse**

Primary infertility
- No previous pregnancy has been achieved

Secondary infertility
- Previous pregnancy has been achieved

Causes of infertility and examples include:
- *Cervical mucus factor*: Refers to poor quality or insufficient mucus, which may arise from infection or hormonal imbalance.
- *Male factor*: Low semen volume, low sperm counts, poor motility and morphology
- *Ovulatory factor*: Anovulatory cycles
- *Peritoneal factor*: Adhesions from prior surgeries, endometriosis, or pelvic inflammatory disease (PID)
- *Uterine-tubal factor*: Anatomical abnormalities such as bicornate uterus, uterine fibroids, cervical stenosis, tubal scarring, or blockage from endometriosis or PID

P **Educate the couple on the optimal window of fertilization**

If female cycles are regular, this would be the 6-day interval before and including the day of ovulation.

Perform investigations for the different causes of infertility if appropriate

Cervical factor
- Postcoital test to evaluate the quality of mucus
  - Positive test should have one mobile sperm per high-power field.
- Treat bacterial infections.
- Refer pt to an infertility specialist for intrauterine insemination.

Male factor
- If semen analysis is abnormal, ask male partner to avoid exposure to extreme temperature, wear loose underwear, and refrain from intercourse for 5 days before the fertile window of ovulation.
- Refer to Urology for removal of varicoceles if detected.

Ovulatory factor
- Basal body temperature charting and progesterone challenge test for those who have oligomenorrhea
- Refer to infertility specialist for clomiphene administration.

Peritoneal factor
- Refer to surgeon for laparoscopic adhesion lysis.

Uterine-tubal factor
- Refer to infertility specialist for hysterosalpingogram, hysteroscopy, or laparoscopy to investigate uterine abnormalities and patency of the fallopian tubes.

Refer for consultation regarding in vitro fertilization if the couple is still unable to conceive
Remind the couple that adoption is an option

S **Does the pt associate the breast pain with any particular event?**
Direct trauma to the breast, increased running, or weightlifting may prompt an episode
of mastalgia.
Pts may describe that mastalgia is associated with the menstrual cycle secondary to the
hormonal influence on the breast tissue.

Has the pt had any nipple discharge?
Lactating women may develop mastitis with associated pus, pain, and fever.

Has the pt found a breast lump in the area of the pain?
Mastalgia can be associated with fibrocystic breasts.

Are there any family members with breast cancer?
First-degree relatives with breast cancer that develops before menopause increases the
pt's risk for breast cancer.

What medications is the pt taking?
Hormone replacement or contraceptives can cause breast pain.

Does the pt have tenderness with deep inspiration?
Chest wall pain and costochondritis can be confused for mastalgia.

O **Perform physical exam**
Chest:
- Perform bilateral breast exam.
- Inspect the breast for any skin changes, bruising, discoloration, erythema, nipple
  retraction, dimpling, or obvious asymmetry.
- Palpate the entire breast area, including the chest wall and axillary areas.
  - Document masses in terms of size, breast, quadrant location, mobility, distance
    from the nipple, and the corresponding time of the clock.
    - Example: 2-cm mobile mass at 11 o'clock, in the upper-outer quadrant of
      the right breast, 5 cm away from the nipple
- Check for reproducible tenderness in any particular area.
- Palpate the sternocostal margins for tenderness, indicating costochondritis.
- Express the nipple for discharge.
  - Guaiac-positive discharge can indicate malignancy.

Consider the following studies:
Mammogram will detect calcifications and is appropriate in women ages 35+ years
and in younger women who are at high risk.
Ultrasound will delineate if a lump is cystic or solid.

A Mastalgia

Cyclic
- Usually bilateral
- Breast pain described as soreness or heaviness.
- May radiate to the axilla
- Worse right before menstruation
- Improves or resolves at the end of menses

Noncyclic
- Unilateral
- Breast pain described as sharp or burning quality.
- Localized to a particular area
- Differential diagnosis of noncyclic mastalgia:
  - Mastitis
  - Malignancy
  - Trauma
  - Costochondritis

P Reassure

Most breast cancers do not present with breast pain.

In up to 80% of pts with breast pain, the pain resolves spontaneously.

Reexamine pt after two menstrual cycles
Check for any palpable abnormalities.

Recommended therapies
Primrose oil
NSAIDs
Support bra
Pain that is severe and unresponsive to conservative therapies may need antigonadotropin therapy with danocrine (refer to Endocrinology).

Other remedies (used but not yet proven to be effective)
Vitamin E
Vitamin B_6
Low-salt diet
Low-caffeine diet

Educate pt on breast self-examination and health maintenance
Breast self-exam should be performed on a monthly basis, during the week after menses.
Stress the importance of screenings and immunizations.

At any point in the workup, if a mass is detected, perform a fine-needle aspiration or refer pt to Surgery for further evaluation

S **What symptoms is the pt experiencing?**
Pt may report depression, difficulty with concentration, hot flashes, insomnia, mood
swings, night sweats, decreased libido, or vaginal dryness.
Irregular menses with associated heavy blood flow may herald perimenopause.

Does the pt have any medical problems?
The use of hormone replacement therapy (HRT) is contraindicated in women with a
history of coronary arery disease (CAD), cerebrovascular accident, liver disease,
venous thrombosis, pulmonary embolism, breast or uterine cancer, or headaches with
focal neurologic symptoms.

Have any family members been diagnosed with breast cancer?
Pts who have first-degree relatives with breast cancer are at a higher risk for breast
cancer and should take this into account when deciding whether to take HRT.

Does the pt smoke?
The use of tobacco and hormones is contraindicated in women ≥ 35 years because of
the increased risk of CAD, stroke, and thrombosis.
Women who smoke are at increased risk of osteoporosis.

O **Perform physical exam**
General: Measure the woman's height to determine if stature is decreasing, indicating
possible osteoporosis.
HEENT: Palpate the neck to check for thyroid masses or nodules.
Breast:
  • Inspect for skin changes, such as thinning or decreased elasticity.
  • Palpate for masses or axillary lymphadenopathy.
Pelvic:
  • Inspection of vaginal vault will show dry, atrophic vaginal walls.
  • There may be pelvic floor laxity, cystocele, or rectocele.
Back: Examine the back for kyphosis or scoliosis.

Consider the following labs and studies:
FSH is elevated.
Estrogen is low.
TSH to rule out thyroid disease
Prolactin to rule out prolactinoma

Menopause
Natural Menopause
- Referred to as "the change"
- Period of time when follicular atresia (depletion of ovarian follicles) results in a drop in estrogen production and cessation in menstruation
- Average age of menopause in the United States is 50 to 52 years.
- Premature ovarian failure is menopause that occurs before the age of 40.

Secondary Menopause
- Surgically induced: Oophorectomy
- Medicinally induced: Antigonadotropins, chemotherapeutics

 Educate pt
Explain to the pt what to expect, including the physiologic, mental, and physical changes that take place.
Provide reading material or websites for the pt to study at home.
Assess the severity of pt's symptoms.
Assess the pt's risks if HRT is a consideration.

Recommend behavioral modification
Dietary changes, daily aerobic exercise, yearly routine health maintenance
Smoking cessation

Consider hormonal versus nonhormonal therapy
Explain the risks of HRT.
Clonidine 0.1 mg po tid for reduction in vasomotor instability
Low-dose SSRIs daily for assistance with vasomotor instability and emotional lability
Natural isoflavones (phytoestrogens) found in soy products and natural progesterone in yam root are helpful in relieving menopausal symptoms.
Estrogen vaginal cream or lubricants for reduction in vaginal dryness
Bisphosphonates or selective estrogen receptor modulator for osteoporosis
Low-dose testosterone injection for decreased libido (review side effect)
HRT can be in pill or patch form.

- Use estrogen alone if pt had a hysterectomy; otherwise, use combination estrogen and progesterone.

Recommend supplements
Calcium 1500 mg with vitamin D 1000 mg po daily
Black cohosh has been shown to mitigate hot flashes.

S **What symptoms is the pt reporting?**

Symptoms of pelvic inflammatory disease (PID) range from subtle lower abdominal pain to severe peritonitis.

Associated symptoms can include nausea, vomiting, fever, abnormal vaginal discharge, or intermittent vaginal bleeding.

When was the pt's last menstrual period?

Gonorrheal infection can begin just after menses.

Does the pt have risk factors for PID?

- Early coitus
- History of sexually transmitted infection (STI)
- Multiple partners
- Symptomatic partner
- No barrier method use
- Prior episode of PID
- IV drug/illicit drug use
- New partner

Has the pt had recent gynecologic instrumentation?

- Endometrial biopsy
- Laparoscopy
- Dilation and curettage
- Hysterosalpingogram
- Intrauterine device placement

O **Check vital signs**

Check for signs of sepsis.

Perform physical exam

General: Pt may appear toxic.
Abdomen:

- Auscultate for bowel sounds.
- Check for masses, rebound, or guarding.

  ◆ Right upper quadrant pain may suggests Fitz-Hugh-Curtis syndrome.

Pelvic:

- Inspect for copious or mucopurulent vaginal discharge.
- Perform bimanual exam to evaluate uterine size.
- Check for cervical motion tenderness.
- Check for adnexal masses or fullness.

Consider the following labs and studies:

UA to rule out urinary tract infection
Urine pregnancy test
Gonorrhea and chlamydia cultures
Abdominal and pelvic ultrasound

A **Pelvic Inflammatory Disease**
Inflammation affecting the female upper genital tract
Minimum criteria for diagnosis includes at least one of the following:
  - Adnexal tenderness
  - Uterine tenderness
  - Cervical motion tenderness
Other supportive criteria:
  - Fever > 101°F
  - Positive gonorrhea or chlamydia culture
  - Abnormal cervical or vaginal discharge
  - Ultrasound with fluid-filled, thickened fallopian tubes
  - Ultrasound with tubo-ovarian complex
  - Ultrasound with free fluid in the pelvis
Causative agents:
          - Chlamydia   - Gonorrhea
          - Gardnerella   - Gram-negative rods (enteric)
          - Anaerobes

P **Start pharmacotherapy in the outpatient setting:**
Quinolone: Levaquin 500 mg po bid _or_ ofloxacin 400 mg po bid
  - Metronidazole 500 mg po bid is to be considered in addition.
  - Duration of treatment is 14 days
Ceftriaxone 250 mg IM single dose _and_ doxycycline 100 mg po bid
  - Metronidazole 500 mg po bid is to be considered in addition.
  - Duration of treatment is 14 days.

Admit pt if:
Pt is unreliable.
Temperature is > 101°F.
Appendicitis is suspected.
Ectopic pregnancy is suspected or uterine pregnancy is discovered.
Tubo-ovarian abscess is suspected.
The pt is unable to tolerate oral intake.
There has been no response within 72 hours of initiating antibiotics.

Evaluate and treat the sexual partner(s) of the infected pt

Educate pt on STIs, safe sexual behavior, and contraceptives

S **Were there any complications with the delivery?**
Eclampsia, endometritis, and hemorrhage are complications that can prolong the
postpartum hospitalization.

Is the pt experiencing any problems?
Typical complaints may include breast pain, constipation, depression, dysuria, fatigue,
and vaginal discharge.

Is the mother breastfeeding or bottle-feeding?
The most common causes of breastfeeding failure include misconceptions about
adequate production, poor positioning techniques, and pain.

Has the pt had pelvic rest since delivery?
No douching, no tampons, and no sexual intercourse are recommended until
postpartum visit

Does the pt have adequate assistance at home?

This is an important time to find out if the mother is feeling fatigued, overwhelmed, or
depressed.

 Perform physical exam
HEENT: Palpate for any thyroid masses or nodules.
Breast:
- Inspect for fissures or bleeding of the nipples.
- Palpate to check for engorgement or masses.
  - ◆ Erythema, increased tenderness, and purulent nipple discharge suggest
    mastitis.
Heart: Audible flow murmur can indicate anemia.
Abdomen: Inspect abdominal wound for healing if pt had a cesarean section.
Pelvic:
- Inspect the external genitalia for lesions or varicosities.
- If episiotomy is present, ensure that the wound is healing.
- Check for any vaginal wall or cervical lesions.
- Palpate uterus and document size.
- Check for foul-smelling lochia or discharge.
Rectum: Inspect for hemorrhoids and ensure that they are not thrombosed.

Consider the following labs and studies:
CBC to check for anemia
Papanicolaou test
Gonorrhea and chlamydia cultures
Vaginal culture if lochia is foul-smelling
Fasting glucose or random glucose testing if the pt had glucose intolerance or
gestational diabetes
Thyroid-stimulating hormone if there were abnormalities during pregnancy

Postpartum Visit
This visit is typically scheduled about 1 month after delivery.

Address the following issues
Anemia
- Prescribe iron sulfate for the pt and recheck CBC in a few weeks.

Breastfeeding
- Encourage breastfeeding.
- Ensure that the pt is not having problems with positioning.
- Explain the safety profile of medications.

Contraception
- Help the pt decide what form of method to use.

Mastitis
- Breast infection will require antibiotics.

Postpartum blues and depression
- Thought to be influenced by the erratic hormonal changes the body undergoes after delivery.
- Postpartum blues are characterized by mood swings taking place within 10 days of delivery and usually resolving on their own.
- Postpartum depression can be preceded by postpartum blues, has onset within the first 3 months, and may require psychotherapy and pharmacotherapy.

Safety
- Emphasize the importance of safety with the arrival of the newborn.
- Dangers of sleeping with the infant in the same bed
- Smoke detectors
- Sibling rivalry
- Tobacco use or second-hand smoke

Social support
- Ensure that the pt has assistance from family members or friends, allowing her to have alone time for herself or for rest.

S **What symptoms of premenstrual syndrome (PMS) or premenstrual dysphoric disorder (PMDD) does the pt report?**

Physical and psychological symptoms:

- Painful cramps/pelvic pain
- Breast tenderness
- Difficulty concentrating
- Depressed mood/mood swing
- Sleep disturbance: Hypersomnia/insomnia
- Strong food cravings/overeating
- Diarrhea

- Headaches
- Bloating
- Hot flushes
- Anxiety
- Fatigue/lethargy
- Crying spells

Symptoms are associated with the menstrual cycle.

Are these symptoms affecting the pt's daily routine or relationships?

Symptoms can be so severe that they disrupt everyday tasks and increase interpersonal conflicts.

Does the pt have any other medical problems?

It is important to exclude medical conditions that PMS/PMDD can mimic:

- Anemia
- Uterine fibroid
- Thyroid disease
- Irritable bowel syndrome

- Endometriosis
- Migraine headaches
- Depression

Have there been any recent stressors?

Stress can exacerbate the symptoms of PMS/PMDD.

O **Perform physical exam**

HEENT: Inspect the thyroid for masses or nodules.

Abdomen: Palpate to exclude any peritoneal signs of rebound or guarding.

Pelvic:

- Inspect the vaginal vault for abnormal discharge to exclude infection.
- Check for cervical motion tenderness.
- Palpate the uterus and adnexa to ensure that there are no masses.

Consider the following labs:

CBC to test for anemia

TSH to rule out thyroid disease

Premenstrual Syndrome
Has a wide spectrum of psychological and physical symptoms described in the "S"
   section.
Symptoms are cyclic and occur during the luteal phase of the menstrual cycle and
   improve at the onset of menses (follicular phase).
Symptoms must be present for at least two consecutive cycles.
Unclear causes are thought to be related to estrogen/progesterone hormonal influence,
   excess prostaglandins, or disruption of the renin-angiotensin-aldosterone system.

Premenstrual Dysphoric Disorder
Psychiatric term used to describe the severe form of PMS
Symptoms affect the pt's daily routine and interpersonal relationships

 Instruct pt to keep a diary of symptoms
This diary should contain the frequency and severity of symptoms along with the
   timing of the menstrual cycle.

Suggest lifestyle modifications
Dietary changes:
  • Increased complex carbohydrates and proteins
  • Decreased caffeine, sodium, and sweets
Increased aerobic exercise at least three times per week
  • Increases the level of circulating endorphins
Stress management and reduction
Vitamin supplements recommended include:
  • Calcium
  • Vitamin E
Vitamin supplements that have been used with less supportive evidence include:
  • Magnesium
  • Vitamin B_6

Start pharmacotherapy
NSAIDs for symptoms of headaches, cramping, and pelvic pain
Oral contraceptive hormones are used to control the level of estrogen and
   progesterone, but their efficacy is unclear.
SSRIs at low doses have shown improvements in symptomatology.
Spironolactone can be used for symptoms of bloating.

S   **Is the pt at risk for sexually transmitted infection (STIs)?**
- Early coitus
- History of STI
- Multiple partners
- Symptomatic partner
- No barrier method use
- Prior episode of pelvic inflammatory disease
- IV drug/illicit drug use
- New partner
- Pts who have used unsterile needles for body piercing, ear piercing, or tattooing can be at risk for STIs.

Has the pt had sexual relations while under the influence of alcohol or drugs?
Alcohol and drugs can impair judgment.

Is the pt having any symptoms suggesting an STI?
Vaginal or urethral discharge, dysuria, and lower abdominal, pelvic, or testicular pain may be presenting symptoms of an STI.

Has the pt noticed skin lesions in the urogenital or anal area?

O   **Perform physical exam**
HEENT: Check for conjunctival discharge (gonorrhea/chlamydia), icteric sclera (hepatitis), or exudates in the throat (gonorrhea/chlamydia).
Abdomen: Palpate for rebound, guarding, or tenderness in lower quadrants.
Urogenital:
- If female, inspect the vulva for any lesions, periurethral abscess, abnormal vaginal discharge, cervical motion tenderness, adnexal masses, or uterine tenderness.
- If male, inspect penis for any lesions, urethral discharge, and epididymal tenderness.
Rectal: Check males for prostate tenderness.
Skin: Inspect for rashes on palms/soles (syphilis), verrucae (genital warts), vesicles (herpes), or ulcerations (herpes/syphilis) on urogenital or perianal skin.
Lymphatics: Palpate for inguinal lymphadenopathy

Consider the following labs and studies:
- HIV
- Papanicolaou test
- Hepatitis B and C serology
- RPR or VDRL
- Herpes simplex viral culture
- Gonorrhea and chlamydia cultures

A   **Sexually Transmitted Infections: Also referred to as sexually transmitted diseases**
Bacterial infections:
- Chlamydia
- Gonorrhea
Viral infections:
- Herpes simplex virus (HSV)
- Hepatitis B and C
- Human immunodeficiency virus (HIV)
- Human papilloma virus (HPV) is responsible for genital warts and cervical cancer.
Protozoan infection:
- *Trichomonas vaginalis*
Treponemal infection:
- Syphilis

P **Identify the causative agent and start appropriate pharmacotherapy**
Treatments listed as follows are primary regimens
Chlamydia
  • Doxycycline 100 mg po bid for 7 days *or*
  • Azithromycin 1 g po single dose
Gonorrhea
  • Ceftriaxone 125 mg IM single dose

  • Treat for both organisms (gonorrhea or chlamydia) if either is detected.
    ◆ A one-time dose of 2 g azithromycin can be used to treat both infections, but
      increased GI side effects may ensue.

Hepatitis B and C
  • Medications approved are interferon, ribavirin, and adefovir, which are usually
    used under the supervision of a specialist.
HSV
  • Dosage and duration of antiviral therapy with acyclovir, famciclovir, or
    valacyclovir depends on whether this is the first episode or not:
    ◆ *First episode*: Acyclovir 400 mg po tid for 7 to 10 days
    ◆ *Recurrent episode*: Acyclovir 400 mg po tid for 5 days
    ◆ *Suppressive therapy*: Acyclovir 400 mg po bid
HIV
  • Antiretrovirals and medical management are provided by an HIV specialist.
HPV
  • Imiquimod, podophyllin, and trichloroacetic acid can all be applied topically.
  • Cryotherapy, electrocautery, or surgical excision can also be used.
Trichomonas vaginalis
  • Metronidazole 2 g po single dose or 500 mg po bid for 5 days
Syphilis
  • Alternatives for penicillin-allergic pts exist but are not listed below.
  • If less than 1 year of infection, treat with penicillin G 2.4 million units IM
  • If more than 1 year of infection or unknown date of contraction, treat with
    penicillin G 2.4 million units IM weekly for 3 weeks

Promote prevention
Immunize for Hepatitis A and B pre-exposure.
Educate about STIs, safe sexual behavior, and contraceptives.
Evaluate and treat the sexual partner(s) of the infected pt.

III

Pediatrics

S **Obtain history from parents**

HPI:

- Address parental concerns.
- Discuss feeding: Breastfeeding versus formula feeding?
  - ◆ Quantity and frequency of feeds
- Discuss elimination and voiding patterns:
  - ◆ How many wet diapers in 24 hours?
  - ◆ How many soiled diapers in 24 hours?
- Discuss sleep patterns and positions.

PMH:

- Prenatal history: Document the number of prenatal care months.
  - ◆ Any exposure to alcohol, tobacco, medications, or drugs?
  - ◆ Any medical problems during pregnancy, such as thyroid disease, anemia, infections, gestational diabetes, eclampsia, or bleeding?
- Birth history: Was the delivery vaginal or cesarean? Forceps or vacuum used?
- Did the baby need to be resuscitated?
- Hospitalization: Did the baby go home with mother or stay for observation?
- Immunizations: Did the baby receive the Hepatitis B vaccine in the hospital?

PSH: Any special procedures:

- If male, was a circumcision performed?

Allergies: Any known drug allergies?

Medications: Is the baby taking any prescribed or over-the-counter medications?

FMH: Review family medical problems, congenital illnesses, or developmental delays.

SH:

- Who are the infant's primary caretakers?
- Number and age of siblings?
- Any exposure to second-hand smoke?
- Are there financial resources to provide for the child?
- Are both parents living together in the same household?

O **Check vital signs**

Fever may warrant a septic workup for a neonatal infection.

Check height, weight, and head circumference charts.

Perform physical exam

General: Observe for any distress.

HEENT:

- Check fontanelles and cranial sutures.
- Examine head for cephalohematomas, craniosynostosis, or hydrocephalus.
- Elicit red reflexes and check for eye discharge.
- Check ear canals and check for any external sinus tracts.
- Examine for a cleft palate, teeth, or thrush on tongue.

Chest: Palpate clavicles for fractures and auscultate breath sounds.

Heart: Listen for the presence of murmurs.

Abdomen:

- Palpate for any abdominal masses.
- Check umbilical cord stump for signs of infection.

Urogenital:

- Inspect for ambiguous genitalia.
- Check urethral meatus for hypospadias in males.

- Palpate testicles if descended; if not, palpate inguinal canals for location.
- Examine for hydroceles, inguinal hernias, and scrotal masses.

Rectum: Look to see if rectum is patent.

Musculoskeletal:
- Perform *Ortolani* and *Barlow* maneuvers for hip dislocation.
- Inspect spine for dimples or hair tufts, which may indicate spina bifida.

Neuro:
- Assess for *Moro*, grasp, and suck reflexes.
- Check hearing grossly by startling with a loud noise.

Skin: Inspect for acne neonatorum, dermal melanocytosis (Mongolian spot), erythema toxicum neonatorum, jaundice, milia, port wine nevus, or facial salmon spot.

Denver developmental assessment of motor, visual, language, and social categories for newborns includes:

- Social smile	- Lifts chin up
- Regards face	- Tracks to midline with eyes

Consider the following labs or follow-up laboratories drawn in the hospital:

Newborn screening test

Blood type/Coombs test for ABO incompatibility

A **Healthy Newborn**

P **Address parental concerns and treat pt if indicated**
Review diet

Feeding on demand: Typically 2 to 3 ounces every 2 to 3 hours

No honey or extra water

Implement prevention

Definition of fever and instruction of what to do:
- If temperature $\geq 100.4°$F rectally, go to the hospital.
- No acetaminophen or aspirin

Discuss Sudden Infant Death Syndrome (SIDS):
- Optimal sleeping position is on the back or the side.

Review safety:

- Parental fatigue	- Second-hand smoke avoidance
- Shaken baby syndrome	- Sibling interaction and bonding
- Smoke detectors	- Water temperature for bathing baby

- Crib safety: Bumpers, bedding, and fire retardant sleepwear
- Car seat: Importance of correct installation and use
  - ◆ Place in center of the back seat, facing rear

Umbilical cord care

Anticipatory guidance:
- Avoid bottle propping
- Symptoms of infant colic

Encourage cardiopulmonary resuscitation (CPR) training

Immunize pt

If Hepatitis B was not given in the hospital, can either be given at this visit or at the 2-month visit.

S **Review each of the categories listed below (Refer to "Newborn Exam" section for specific questions in each of the categories.)**

HPI:

- Address parental concerns.
- Did the infant have any reaction to immunization given at last visit?
- Has the infant had any recent illness?
- Ask about diet and dietary habits: Timing of feeds or meals.
- What are the infant's elimination and voiding patterns?
- Inquire about sleeping patterns: Hours of continuous sleep and daytime naps.
- Has the infant had any accidents?

PMH: Review Prenatal History and Birth History (See Newborn Exam p. 98)

- Hospitalization: Any emergency room visits or hospitalizations?
- Immunizations: Are any immunizations missing?

PSH: Any surgeries or special procedures since last visit?

Allergies: Any known drug allergies?

Medications: Using prescribed or over-the-counter medications?

FMH: See Newborn Exam (p. 98)

SH

- Any changes in family dynamics?
- Are both parents involved in the care of the infant?
- Who are the caregivers? Any babysitters?
- Are both parents employed outside of the home?

O **Check vital signs**

Fever may warrant a septic workup for an infection.

Check height, weight, and head circumference charts for age-appropriate growth.

Perform physical exam

General: Inspect for signs of abuse or neglect.

HEENT:

- Examine fontanelles.
- Check for red reflex and strabismus.
- Visualize tympanic membranes.
- Look for teeth eruptions, nasal polyps, or neck masses.

Lymphatics: Palpate for lymphadenopathy.

Chest: Auscultate for wheezing, crackles, or ronchi.

Heart: Listen for a murmur.

Abdomen: Palpate for masses or umbilical hernias.

Urogenital:

- Inspect for abnormal findings.
- If male, palpate for descended testicles or scrotal masses.

Musculoskeletal: Check for hip clicks and bowing of legs.

Skin: Inspect for rashes, nevi, or growths.

Neuro: Check cranial nerves and muscular tone.

Reflexes: Age at which specific reflexes disappear:

- *Moro*/stepping by 2 months	- Rooting by 4 months
- Palmar grasp by 6 months	- Plantar grasp by 9 to 12 months

Denver Developmental Assessment:

2 Months: Holds head, follows past midline, squeals

4 Months: Able to roll front to back and grasp with hands together, sits while propped up, turns toward voice, can "coo"

6 Months: Rolls from back to front, sits without support, rakes and transfers objects between hands, babbles mama/dada (nonspecific)

9 Months: Crawls, pulls to stand, uses pincer grasp, finger feeds, holds bottle, babbles mama/dada (specific)

12 Months: If not walking, may cruise with furniture or stand, uses mature pincer grasp, drinks from a cup, follows one-step commands, speaks words

Consider obtaining the following labs:
CBC or hemoglobin/hematocrit (9 to 12 months) for anemia
Lead level (12 months) for lead poisoning

A Well Child Exam (2–12 Months)

P **Address parental concerns and treat pt if indicated**
Review diet
Discuss age-appropriate diets.
Review when to start juices, rice cereals, and solids.
Discuss appropriate portions.
Switch to whole milk with vitamin D at 12 months.

Implement prevention
Definition of fever and instruction on what to do:
- Temperature $\geq 100.4°$F rectally (Rectal temperature is higher than axillary, oral, and tympanic temperatures.)
- Review appropriate dose of acetaminophen or ibuprofen.

Review safety: (Refer to safety issues in "Newborn Exam" section.)
Additional topics include:
- Child-proofing the house: Cabinet locks, electrical outlet covers, keeping drugs or chemicals out of reach, window locks, guards for stairways
- Give Poison Control telephone number.
- Dangers of walkers
- Gun safety: If gun is in home, keep it locked and out of reach.

Anticipatory guidance: Dental care, stranger anxiety, and separation anxiety

Immunize pt
Give appropriate immunizations for age.
See Centers for Disease Control and Prevention (CDC) website for an updated schedule: *www.cdc.gov/nip*

S **Review each of the categories listed below (Refer to Newborn Exam p. 98 section for specific questions in each of the categories.)**
HPI:
- Address parental concerns.
- Did the pt have any reaction to immunizations given at last visit?
- Has the pt had any recent illness?
- Ask about diet and dietary habits: Timing of feeds or meals.
- What are the pt's elimination and voiding patterns?
- Inquire about sleeping patterns: Hours of continuous sleep and daytime naps.
- Has the pt had any accidents?
- Does the pt attend daycare?

PMH: Review Prenatal History and Birth History (See Newborn Exam p. 98)
- Hospitalization: Any emergency room visits or hospitalizations?
- Immunizations: Are any immunizations missing?

PSH: Any surgeries or special procedures since last visit?
Allergies: Any known drug allergies?
Medications: Using prescribed or over-the-counter medications?
FMH and SH: See Newborn Exam p. 98

O **Check vital signs**
Check height, weight, and head circumference charts for age-appropriate growth.
- Monitor for disproportionate or accelerated weight gain or loss.

Perform physical exam
General: Inspect for signs of abuse or neglect.
HEENT:
- Examine fontanelles.
- Check for red reflex and strabismus.
- Visualize tympanic membranes.
- Look for teeth eruptions or decay.

Lymphatics: Palpate for lymphadenopathy.
Chest: Auscultate for wheezing, crackles, or ronchi.
Heart: Listen for a murmur.
Abdomen: Palpate for masses or umbilical hernias.
Urogenital:
- Inspect for abnormal findings.
- If male, palpate for descended testicles or scrotal masses.

Musculoskeletal:
- Check for hip clicks and bowing of legs.
- Inspect back and joints.

Skin: Inspect for rashes, nevi, or growths.
Neuro: Assess cranial nerves, strength, sensory, reflexes, and gait.

Denver developmental assessment:
15 Months: Walks alone, backwards and upstairs, scribbles, points to body parts, uses spoon, speaks five words, indicates wants
18 Months: Runs, throws overhand, kicks ball forward, removes clothing, speaks 10 to 20 words
24 Months: Can wash and dry hands, remove clothing, walk up and down stairs, jump up, open doors, combine two to three words

Consider the following labs:
CBC or hemoglobin/hematocrit
Lead level (24 months)

 Well Child Exam (13–24 Months)

 Address parental concerns and treat pt if indicated
Review diet
Discuss age-appropriate diets.
Discuss appropriate portions.
Switch to low-fat or nonfat milk with vitamin D at 24 months.

Implement prevention
Definition of fever and instruction on what to do:
- Temperature ≥100.4°F rectally (Rectal temperature is higher than axillary, oral, and tympanic temperatures.)
- Review appropriate dose of acetaminophen or ibuprofen.

Review safety: (Refer to safety issues in Newborn Exam p. 98)
Additional topics include:
- Limit television viewing and exposure to violence.

Anticipatory guidance:
- Dental care	- Picky eating
- Promote reading	- Toilet training between 15 to 36 months
- Frequent viral illnesses (especially if in daycare)	

Immunize pt
Give appropriate immunizations for age.
See Centers for Disease Control and Prevention (CDC) website for an updated
schedule: *www.cdc.gov/nip*

S **Review each of the categories listed below (Refer to Newborn Exam p. 98 for specific questions in each of the categories.)**

HPI:

- Address parental concerns.
- Did the pt have any reaction to immunizations given at last visit?
- Has the pt had any recent illness?
- Ask about diet and dietary habits: Timing of feeds or meals.
- What are the pt's elimination or voiding patterns?
- Inquire about sleep patterns: Hours of continuous sleep and daytime naps.
- How many hours does the pt spend watching television, listening to the radio, playing video games, or playing on the computer?
- Has the pt had any accidents?
- Does the pt attend daycare or school?
- If the pt is in school, how is he or she performing?
- Is the child participating in extracurricular activities or organized sports?
- Are there any behavioral issues or misconduct?
- If female, has the pt started her menses?

PMH: Review Prenatal History and Birth History (See Newborn Exam p. 98)

- Hospitalizations: Any emergency room visits or hospitalizations?
- Immunizations: Are any immunizations missing?

PSH: Any surgeries or special procedures since last visit?

Allergies: Any known drug allergies?

Medications: Using prescribed or over-the-counter medications?

FMH and SH: See Newborn Exam (p. 98)

O **Check vital signs**

Check height, weight, and head circumference charts for age-appropriate growth.

- Monitor for disproportionate or accelerated weight gain or loss.

Perform physical exam

General: Inspect for signs of abuse or neglect.

HEENT:

- Check for red reflex and strabismus.
- Visualize tympanic membranes.
- Look for teeth eruptions or decay.

Lymphatics: Palpate for lymphadenopathy.

Chest: Auscultate for wheezing, crackles, or ronchi.

Heart: Listen for a murmur.

Abdomen: Palpate for masses or umbilical hernias.

Urogenital:

- Inspect for abnormal findings.
- If male, palpate for descended testicles or scrotal masses.
- Check that foreskin, if present, is retractable.

Musculoskeletal: Examine for scoliosis or joint laxity.

Skin: Inspect for rashes, nevi, or growths.

Neuro: Assess cranial nerves, strength, sensory, reflexes, and gait.

Denver developmental assessment:

30 Months: Copies a vertical line, balances on one foot for one second

3 Years: Copies a circle, pedals a tricycle, knows first and last names, dresses with supervision

4 Years: Copies a square, draws a person with three parts, catches a ball, hops on one foot, dresses without supervision

5 Years: Copies a triangle, draws a person with six parts, distinguishes left from right, walks heel to toe

Consider the following labs and studies:

CBC or hemoglobin/hematocrit for anemia

Lead level if at risk for exposure or no prior lead level obtained

UA for proteinuria, glucosuria, hematuria, or infection

Snellen for visual acuity

Audiogram for hearing

A **Well Child Exam (25 Months–Preadolescence)**

P **Address parental concerns and treat pt if indicated**
Review diet

Discuss age-appropriate diets.

Discuss appropriate portions.

Limit junk food.

Implement prevention

Definition of fever and instruction on what to do:

- Temperature ≥ 100.4°F rectally (Rectal temperature is higher than axillary, oral, and tympanic temperatures.)
- Review appropriate dose of acetaminophen or ibuprofen.

Review safety: (Refer to safety issues in Newborn Exam p. 98 section.)

Additional topics include:

- Limit time for television, video games, and computers.
- Prevent exposure to violence in television, video games, and Internet.

Anticipatory guidance: Dental care, picky eating, toilet training between 15 to 36 months; promote reading and exercise; frequent viral illnesses

Immunize pt

Give appropriate immunizations for age.

See Centers for Disease Control and Prevention (CDC) website for an updated schedule: *www.cdc.gov/nip*

S **Review each of the categories listed below (Refer to Newborn Exam p. 98 for specific questions in each of the categories.)**

HPI: Address parental concerns.

PMH: Review Prenatal History and Birth History (See Newborn Exam p. 98)
- Hospitalization: Emergency room visits or hospitalizations?
- Immunizations: Are any immunizations missing?

PSH: Surgeries or special procedures since last visit?

Allergies: Any known drug allergies?

Medications: Using prescribed or over-the-counter medications?

FH: See Newborn Exam p. 98

SH: *HEADSSS assessment for adolescent pts*
- <u>H</u>ome: Review relationship with parents, family members, and general home life.
- <u>E</u>ducation: How is the school performance? Good or bad grades? Any problems?
- <u>A</u>ctivities: Inquire about hobbies, after-school activities, interests, sports, music preferences, friends, and involvement in gangs.
  - How many hours does the pt spend watching television, listening to the radio, playing video games, playing on the computer, or talking on the phone?
- <u>D</u>rugs and <u>D</u>iet
  - Has the teenager had exposure to alcohol, tobacco, or drugs?
  - What does the daily diet consist of?
- <u>S</u>exuality: Is the teenager currently in a relationship? Attracted to the opposite sex or same sex? Has the pt had sexual intercourse? How many partners? Exposure to sexually transmitted infections? Contraceptive method?
- <u>S</u>uicide: Has the teenager contemplated or attempted suicide in the past? Is the teenager depressed?
- <u>S</u>afety: Ask about the use of seatbelts, helmets, and guns. Exposure to abuse or violence? Has the pt had any accidents?

Ob/Gyn:
- Menarche, last menstrual period, frequency, duration, and dysmenorrhea?
- Last Pap test? Any abnormalities? Sexually transmitted infections?
- Any pregnancies?

O **Check vital signs**
Check height, weight, and body mass index.

Perform physical exam

General: Inspect for signs of abuse or neglect.

HEENT:
- Check pupils for size, shape, reactivity to light, and accommodation.
- Visualize tympanic membranes.
- Look for tooth decay or gingivitis.

Lymphatics: Palpate for lymphadenopathy.

Chest:
- Auscultate for wheezing, crackles, or ronchi.
- Perform breast exam and *Tanner stage* if female.

Heart: Listen for a murmur.

Abdomen: Palpate for masses or umbilical hernias.

Urogenital:
- Inspect for lesions and *Tanner stage.*
- If male, palpate for descended testicles or scrotal masses.
- If female, inspect external genitalia and perform pelvic exam if indicated.

Musculoskeletal: Examine for scoliosis or joint laxity.
Skin: *Inspect for acne, tattoos, piercings,* rashes, nevi, or growths.
Neuro: Assess cranial nerves, strength, sensory, reflexes, and gait.

Consider the following labs and studies:
CBC
UA
Snellen and audiogram
If the teen is sexually active, perform the following:
- Papanicolaou test	- Gonorrhea and chlamydia cultures
- Syphilis	- Hepatitis B and C serology
- HIV	

Well Child Exam (Adolescence)

Address parental concerns and treat pt if indicated
Review diet
Discuss dietary intake and appropriate portions.
Limit junk food.

Implement prevention
Review safety:
- Give telephone number of a 24-hour information hotline:
  - Suicide hotline, family planning, peer counseling
- Gun safety: No playing with guns whether loaded or not
- Limit time for television, video games, and computers.
- Prevent exposure to violence on television, video games, and Internet.
  - Dangers of chat rooms

If any problems or high-risk behaviors identified in HEADSSS assessment, make appropriate referrals or interventions.
Discuss safe sex and emergency contraception.
Anticipatory guidance: Promote dental care, reading, and exercise.

Immunize pt
Give appropriate immunizations for age.
See Centers for Disease Control and Prevention (CDC) website for an updated schedule: *www.cdc.gov/nip*

S **When did the abdominal pain begin?**
The chances of a gastrointestinal infection are high if there has been recent travel outside the country, ingestion of contaminated water or food, recent sick contacts, or fever.
Inquire about pain following any recent abdominal trauma.

What are the characteristics of the abdominal pain?
Information regarding the quality, duration, location, and radiation of the pain can yield important clues that will help determine the primary cause.

Is the pt tolerating liquids or solids?
Intractable vomiting and diarrhea can result in dehydration.

Does the pt have any medical conditions?
Pts with sickle cell disease, diabetes mellitus, biliary disease, or peptic ulcers can present with severe abdominal pain.

Has the pt been sexually active?
Both pelvic inflammatory disease and ectopic pregnancy can cause abdominal pain.

O **Check vital signs**
Check for fever and signs of hemodynamic instability.
Height/weight charts: Check for weight loss and deceleration of growth curve.

Perform physical exam
General: Observe for facial grimacing, crying, and restlessness during the exam.
HEENT: Inspect mucous membranes and fontanelles (if present) for signs of dehydration.
Chest:
- Auscultate lung fields for crackles, ronchi, or decreased breath sounds.
- Lower lobe pneumonias can present as abdominal pain.
Abdomen:
- Observe for abdominal distention and for signs of rebound or guarding, which may indicate peritoneal irritation.
- *McBurney point*: Point of maximum tenderness to palpation about one-third away from the anterosuperior iliac spine to the umbilicus
- *Rovsing's sign*: When palpation in the lower left quardrant elicits pain in the right lower quadrant
- *Obturator sign*: Pain with internal rotation of flexed hip and knee
- *Psoas sign*: Pain that can be elicited with full extension of the hip and knee or with lifting the thigh against pressure
- *Murphy's sign*: Pain in the right upper quadrant that halts inspiration upon palpation
- Assess the quality of the bowel sounds, if present.
Back: Check for costovertebral angle tenderness.
Urogenital:
- Examine for hernias.
- If male, palpate the testicles for tenderness.
- If female and sexually active, check for abnormal discharge, cervical motion tenderness, adnexal masses, or uterine enlargement.
Rectal: Inspect for anal fissures or hard stool in vault.

Consider the following labs or studies:
CBC to check for leukocytosis
Chemistry panel to check for dehydration (low bicarbonate level)
UA to rule out UTI
LFT/amylase/lipase to rule out biliary disease, pancreatitis, or ruptured bowel
Stool studies are indicated if there is a history of diarrhea
Urine pregnancy test
Abdominal x-ray series/ultrasound/CT scan as indicated based on exam

Abdominal Pain
The most important thing is to rule out acute abdomen:

- Always rule out appendicitis.

The age group of the pt also helps in determining the most likely cause.
Although the differential diagnosis list is extensive, "VITAMIN C" can allow you to
recall different causes:

- _Vascular_: Henoch-Schönlein purpura, sickle cell crisis
- _Infections_: Appendicitis, cholecystitis, gastroenteritis, mesenteric adenitis,
  pneumonia (lower lobe), peptic ulcer disease, pelvic inflammatory disease,
  tubo-ovarian abscess, UTI
- _Trauma/Tumor_: Foreign body; liver, kidney, or spleen laceration; neuroblastoma,
  Wilms' tumor
- _Anatomic_: Adhesions, bezoar, constipation, ectopic pregnancy, hernia,
  Hirschsprung's disease, intussusception, malrotation, testicular torsion, volvulus
- _Metabolic/Medications_: Antibiotics, diabetic ketoacidosis, lactose intolerance,
  porphyria, NSAIDs
- _Inflammatory_: Esophagitis, gastritis, inflammatory bowel disease
- _Neurologic (Psychiatric)_: Anxiety, depression, and school phobia
- _Colic_

Admit pts presenting with an acute abdomen
Surgical consult must be obtained emergently.

Treat abdominal pain after diagnosing the underlying cause
Obtain appropriate referrals based on suspicion.

S **What signs and symptoms of acute gastroenteritis (AGE) does the pt report?**

Pts may complain of the sudden onset of loose, watery, voluminous, or frequent bowel movements.

Diarrhea may have associated symptoms of abdominal cramping, pain, fever, nausea, vomiting, concentrated urine, or decreased urine production.

Were the symptoms precipitated by a particular food?

It is important to review all foods consumed 24 hours before the onset of illness.

- New foods
- Foods prepared outside of home

Symptoms of diarrhea occur after the consumption of milk or dairy products in pts with lactose intolerance.

Are there any other contacts with similar symptoms?

Household members or daycare members may have infected the pt.

Is the pt tolerating liquids or solids?

Intractable vomiting and diarrhea can result in dehydration.

Is the pt taking any medications?

Antibiotics, milk of magnesia, and laxatives can all cause loose stools.

O **Check vital signs**

Check for fever and signs of hemodynamic instability.

Perform physical exam

General: Ensure that the pt is not lethargic or obtunded.

HEENT:

- Check tympanic membranes for signs of infection because otitis media can present with vomiting.
- Inspect mucous membranes and fontanelles (if present) for dehydration.
  - ◆ Sunken fontanelle and orbits are signs of dehydration.

Heart: Auscultate for tachycardia, and check for delay in capillary refill.

Abdomen:

- Assess the quality of the bowel sounds, if present.
- Palpate for any masses, tenderness, rebound, or guarding.
  - ◆ AGE usually has diffused tenderness.

Urogenital: If pt is still in diapers, check contents for urine and stool.

Skin: Check for decreased skin turgor, cool temperature, or mottled appearance.

Consider the following labs and studies:

CBC to check for leukocytosis

UA to rule out UTI

Chemistry panel to check for dehydration (low bicarbonate level)

Stool studies are indicated if there is a history of diarrhea.

- Stool leukocytes, stool culture, ova, and parasites

Additional stool studies: *Clostridium difficile* toxin, Rotazyme assay

Consider abdominal x-ray series if obstruction or perforation is suspected.

Acute Gastroenteritis
Common bacterial causes associated with bloody diarrhea:

- *Campylobacter jejuni*   - *Clostridium difficile*
- *Escherichia coli*   - *Salmonella*
- *Shigella*   - *Yersinia enterocolitica*

Common bacterial causes associated with toxin-mediated diarrhea:

- *Staphylococcus aureus*   - *Bacillus cereus*
- *Clostridium perfringes*

Common viral causes:

- Adenovirus   - Astrovirus
- Norwalk virus   - Rotavirus

Common parasitic causes:

- *Blastocystis hominis*   - *Cryptosporidium parvum*
- *Entamoeba histolytica*   - *Giardia lambia*
- *Strongyloides stercoralis*

Other causes of diarrhea:

- Inflammatory bowel disease   - Intussusception
- Lactose intolerance   - Stool impaction

Emphasize hydration with oral rehydration solutions:
If the pt is unable to tolerate liquids, admission is warranted for IV fluids.
Start age-appropriate diet as tolerated.
Antiemetics and antidiarrheal medications are not indicated.

Identify the underlying cause of diarrhea:
If a bacterial or parasitic cause is identified, then specific antimicrobials may be
    prescribed.
Inflammatory bowel disease may require endoscopy with biopsy.
Intussusception may need an enema for attempted reduction; however, failure will
    require surgical intervention with resection.
Lactose intolerance responds well to a lactose-free diet.
Stool impaction that is causing overflow diarrhea may require enemas for disimpaction.

Educate on prevention:
Frequent hand washing is encouraged to prevent reinfection or spread of any infectious
    agent.

S

What symptoms is the pt experiencing?

- Ear pain	- Fever	- Otorrhea
- Hearing loss	- Vomiting	- Pulling of the ears
- Upper respiratory infection (URI)		

Was the pt born with a cleft palate or other facial abnormality?
These pts have an increased risk of infection.

Is the pt bottle-feeding?
Bottle propping can lead to ear infections.

Does the pt attend a daycare or have young siblings at home?
These children are at risk for multiple URIs.

Is the pt exposed to second-hand smoke?
Smoke increases the risk of developing ear infections.

Has there been any trauma to the ear that could lead to infection?

- Bite	- Scratch	- Cotton swab use
- Diving	- Flying	- Swimming

Have there been recent or prior episodes of ear pain or infection?

Identifying possible treatment failures assists in choosing the appropriate antibiotics.

O

Check vital signs
Check for fever.

Perform physical exam
HEENT:
- Inspect the pinna and ear canal for erythema or swelling.
- Tenderness elicited with movement of the ear's tragus suggests otitis externa.
- Check the canal for blood, cerumen impaction, discharge, or foreign object.
- Inspect tympanic membranes for bulging, erythema, opacity, distorted landmarks, or perforation, suggesting otitis media.
- Check the mobility of the tympanic membrane using pneumatic otoscopy via insufflation or tympanometry.
  - ◆ Decreased mobility in otitis media and with middle ear effusion
- Check for nasal secretions and enlarged tonsils.
- Palpate the periauricular areas for lymphadenopathy and mastoiditis.

Consider the following labs:
Usually unnecessary
- Consider Gram stain and culture if discharge is present in canal.
- Tympanocentesis may be obtained to determine the cause if pt has failed first- and second-line treatment or if pt is a neonate.

Acute Otitis Media is defined as inflammation in the middle ear, behind the tympanic membrane
Common bacterial causes:
- *Streptococcus pneumoniae*
- *Moraxella catarrhalis*
- *Haemophilus influenzae*
- Group A streptococcus

Common viral causes:
- Respiratory syncytial virus
- Parainfluenza
- Rhinovirus
- Influenza A
- Adenovirus

Otitis Externa is defined as inflammation involving the outer ear, in front of the tympanic membrane: ear canal, meatus, and/or pinna
Can exist with otitis media, especially if the tympanic membrane has perforated
Common bacterial causes:
- *Pseudomonas aeruginosa*
- *Staphylococcus aureus*
- *Proteus mirabilus*
- *Klebsiella pneumoniae*
- *Staphylococcus epidermidis*

Less common causes:
- Herpes virus
- Fungi

P **Treat Acute Otitis Media with oral antibiotic and analgesics**
Amoxicillin: Regular dose: 40 mg/kg/day
- High dose: 80 mg/kg/day
- If failure, consider amoxicillin/clavulanate acid
Cephalosporins (second generation): Cefuroxime, ceftriaxone
Macrolides: Azithromycin, erythromycin/sulfisoxazole
Analgesia with acetaminophen, ibuprofen, or topical anesthetic eardrops

Surgical intervention requires myringotomy and tympanostomy tube placement
Necessary in cases involving recurrent infections or persistent middle ear effusion

Treat Otitis Externa by:
Removing any foreign bodies
Prescribing topical and systemic antibiotics in cases with cellulitis
- If perforation is seen or suspected, use suspension eardrops instead of solution.
Prescribing analgesics (see Acute Otitis Media section)

Surgical intervention may be necessary if abscess is present
Recommend dry ear precautions when showering or swimming
Use a blow dryer to decrease moisture in ear canal.
Wear earplugs to keep the water out.
Use acetic acid eardrops.

S **Does the pt present with symptoms of hyperactivity?**
Fidgeting with hands or feet
Squirming in the seat/restless
Talking excessively
Difficulty engaging in quiet activities
Always "on the go"
Danger of harming self: Runs/climbs in inappropriate situations
Out of seat when inappropriate, or without permission

Does the pt present with symptoms of impulsivity?
Difficulty waiting turn
Interrupting or intruding on others

Does the pt present with symptoms of inattention?
Always losing things
Difficulty organizing activities
Unable to follow instructions
Fails to pay attention to detail
Forgetful and easily distracted:
  • Appears to be daydreaming or not to be listening when spoken to
  • Reluctant to participate in tasks requiring sustained mental effort
  • Difficulty sustaining attention when participating in tasks

Does the child have school or academic difficulties?
Children are usually identified as having attention-deficit/hyperactivity disorder
  (ADHD) when they are of school age and fail to perform as well as their peers.

Does the pt have other behavioral conditions?
Anxiety disorder, conduct disorder, depressive disorder, and oppositional defiant
  disorder can be present in pts with ADHD.

Review prenatal, birth, and past medical history
Exposure to illicit drugs during prenatal period has been associated with ADHD.

Did any particular event prompt the behavior?
Recent unstable home environment or tragic events around the time the symptoms
  began can suggest another cause for the pt's behavior.

O **Perform physical exam**
Physical exam is usually normal except for the following:
  • General: Pt may be very restless or fidgety.
  • Neuro: Perform a thorough neurologic exam, which may only have subtle
    findings.
    ◆ Dysdiadochokinesia may be present (usually seen in cerebellar problems).
      • Rapid alternating hand movements are slow, clumsy, or irregular.

Consider the following studies:
Audiogram to rule out hearing loss
Snellen eye exam to rule out visual impairment

Attention-Deficit/Hyperactivity Disorder
Cause is not completely known, but symptoms are "maladaptive and inconsistent" for the pt's level of development.
Diagnosis depends on fulfilling the criteria listed in the Diagnostic and Statistical Manual of Mental Disorder (DSM-IV criteria can be found in "S" section on p. 114):
  • Pt must have at least six of the symptoms listed under "hyperactivity" and "impulsivity."
  • Pt must have at least six of the symptoms listed under "inattention."
  • Symptoms must have begun before 7 years of age.
  • Symptoms are present in more than one setting (school and home).
  • Symptoms of inattention have been present for at least 6 months.
  • Symptoms are causing significant impairment in academic, occupational, or social aspects.
  • Symptoms are not accounted for by an underlying developmental disorder, schizophrenia, psychotic disorder, or another mental disorder.
Standardized behavioral checklists can be used as tools for diagnosing ADHD.
Evaluation should include assessment for behavioral comorbid conditions.

 Recommend modification of behavior
Getting organized, avoiding procrastination, and completing one project before starting another are some changes the pt can make.
Refer to a child psychiatrist
Start pharmacotherapy
Short-acting
  • Methylphenidate (Ritalin), dextroamphetamine (Dexedrine)
Long-acting
  • Ritalin SR, Metadate ER, Dexedrine Spansules, and pemoline (Cylert)
Combination of rapid onset and long duration:
  • Methylphenidate (Concerta) and combination amphetamine and dextroamphetamine (Adderall)
Antidepressants:
  • Tricyclic antidepressants, SSRIs, and buproprion
Antihypertensives:
  • α_2 blockers

Review side effects of medications during each visit and monitor pt's weight
Educate the family members about ADHD and provide local listing of support groups

S **Are there any symptoms associated with the fever?**
Nausea, vomiting, diarrhea, irritability, cough, rash, rhinorrhea (runny nose), sore
  throat, abdominal pain, or ear pain can all be associated with fever.

How was the temperature measured?
Rectal measurements are the best way to obtain the body's core temperature.

Has the pt had any sick contacts?
Pts attending daycare or living with young siblings are prone to upper respiratory
  infection.

Is the pt tolerating liquids?
Fever increases insensible losses, which can promote dehydration unless the pt is able to
  keep up with hydration.

Does the pt have a significant past medical history?
Gathering information regarding prenatal and birth period, prior hospitalizations, and
  any recent illness can lead to clues as to the possible diagnosis.

O **Check vital signs**
Check to see if pt is hemodynamically stable.

Perform physical exam
General: Observe pt's overall state.
  • Pt may be active and alert versus irritable, inconsolable, or lethargic.
HEENT:
  • If fontanelle is present, check if it is bulging or depressed.
  • Check eyes for mucous discharge, suggesting conjunctivitis.
  • Inspect tympanic membranes for erythema or bulging.
  • Check for mucopurulent nasal discharge with facial tenderness, suggesting
    sinusitis.
  • Ensure that the mucous membranes are moist.
  • If teeth are present, check for cavities or gingival swelling, suggesting possible
    abscess.
  • Look for tonsillar exudates or erythema, suggesting tonsillitis.
Heart: Auscultate for the presence of tachycardia and flow murmur.
Chest: Assess the lungs for the presence of pneumonia or bronchiolitis by listening for
  crackles, egophony, ronchi, or wheezing.
Abdomen:
  • Assess the quality of the bowel sounds, if present.
  • Check for peritoneal signs of rebound or guarding.
Musculoskeletal:
  • Inspect all joints for erythema or swelling.
  • Pts who have a septic joint may refuse to move it or bear weight.
Skin: Inspect for ecchymosis, macules, papules, petechia, or vesicles.
Neuro: Check for meningeal signs: nuchal rigidity, *Kernig's sign*, or *Brudzinski sign*

Consider the following labs and studies:

- CBC	- Blood cultures
- UA	- CXR
- Lumbar puncture	- Stool studies

Fever

Defined as temperature $\geq 100.4°\mathrm{F}$

May be secondary to infection, inflammation, ingestion, malignancy

Determine which pts are high-risk, requiring hospitalization:
- No identifiable source and less than 90 days of life
- WBCs less than 5,000 mm^3 or greater than 15,000 mm^3
- Bandemia ("Left shift")
- History of chronic illness
- History of prematurity
- Recent hospitalization
- Failed outpatient antibiotic treatment
- Not tolerating oral intake

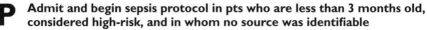 **Admit and begin sepsis protocol in pts who are less than 3 months old, considered high-risk, and in whom no source was identifiable**

Start empiric IV antibiotic therapy.

Obtain all cultures before starting antibiotics.

Start IV fluids for dehydration caused by sensible and insensible losses.

Order acetaminophen or ibuprofen for fever control.

Begin outpatient treatment if a source is identified, the pt is at least 3 months old, and pt is not considered high-risk

Review with the parents the dosage, frequency, and total duration of the antibiotic.

Review the dosage and frequency of the antipyretic adequate for the weight of the pt.

Counsel the parents regarding warning signs and symptoms indicative of deteriorating health.

Schedule a follow-up appointment in the next 24 to 48 hours.

S **Does the pt have any difficulties with breathing?**

Labored breathing can suggest heart abnormality:
- Episodic perioral cyanosis (bluish discoloration around the mouth)
- Nasal flaring
- Neck or chest retractions
- Abdominal retractions
- Orthopnea (dyspnea when lying down)

Is the pt experiencing any difficulty with feeding?

Difficulty feeding as a result of a heart abnormality can result in failure to thrive:
- Choking   - Coughing
- Diaphoresis   - Gagging with feeds

Has the pt had limited exercise tolerance?

Pts with certain heart murmurs may experience chest pain, near-syncope, or syncopal events.

Was there drug exposure during the perinatal period?

Alcohol exposure can lead to fetal alcohol syndrome, which is associated with atrial and ventricular septal defects.

O **Check vital signs**

Compare upper extremity blood pressure to lower extremity: usually 10 mm Hg higher in the lower extremity.
- If the same or lower, suspect coarctation of the aorta.

Height/weight curve: Failure to thrive

Perform physical exam

HEENT: Inspect for jugular venous distention, which is seen in heart failure.

Chest: Assure that the pt has clear lung fields.
- Crackles can indicate heart failure.

Heart:
- Describe the quality and the location of the murmur.
    - Timing: Systolic versus diastolic versus holosystolic
- Auscultate for clicks, gallops, trills, or radiation of murmur.
    - S_3 may be heard with mitral or tricuspid regurgitation.
    - S_4 may be heard in aortic stenosis, pulmonary hypertension, and pulmonary stenosis.
- Palpate chest wall for the point of maximal impulse.
    - Displaced when the heart is enlarged

Extremities:
- Check pulses in upper and lower extremities.
    - Bounding versus diminished
- Inspect nail beds for cyanosis.
- Check for pedal edema.

Consider the following labs and studies:

CBC to rule out anemia

ECG

CXR

Heart Murmur (Types)
Functional:
- *Pulmonary flow murmur*: High-pitched blowing
- *Still's murmur*: Vibratory quality
- *Venous hum*: Continuous soft humming

Congenital heart lesions:
- *Aortic stenosis*: Crescendo-decrescendo, high-pitched
- *Atrial septal defect (ASD)*: Medium-pitched systolic ejection
- *Coarctation of the aorta*: Systolic ejection click of bicuspid aortic valve, disparity with bounding upper extremity pulses, and weak lower pulses
- *Patent ductus arteriosus (PDA)*: Continuous machine-like
- *Pulmonic stenosis*: Crescendo-decrescendo, low-pitched
- *Ventricular septal defect (VSD)*: If small VSD, loud and harsh blowing; if large VSD, then soft blowing

Physiologic murmurs:
- High cardiac output
  - Anemia
  - Hyperthyroidism

 Reassure parents about functional or physiologic murmurs
Functional murmurs do not require intervention and disappear.

Observe and schedule follow-up appointments
Sometimes an ASD, VSD, or PDA may spontaneously close.

Refer to Cardiology
Not all murmurs require echocardiogram.
Some murmurs do need to be followed by a cardiologist to ensure that there is no worsening, leading to congestive heart failure.
- Pt may need cardiac catheterization to evaluate heart function and the extent of a lesion.
- If murmur is severe, pt may be referred to cardiothoracic surgeon for repair or valve replacement.

S **When did the symptoms start?**

Most children achieve nighttime bladder control by the age of 5 years.

Does the pt have any daytime urinary voiding dysfunctions?
These symptoms suggest another diagnosis, not nocturnal enuresis:
- Dribbling   - Dysuria
- Frequency   - Hesitancy
- Straining   - Weak stream
- Urgency   - Urine loss

Does the pt have a significant past medical history?
Conditions such as diabetes insipidus, diabetes mellitus, developmental delay, seizures, and sleep apnea are all causes of urinary incontinence.
Surgeries or injuries to the genital area or back can be responsible for enuresis.

Is the pt having a problem with constipation or stool incontinence?
The presence of constipation, stool incontinence, and enuresis should prompt investigation of the spinal cord.

Has the pt had any recent stressors, trauma, or changes coinciding with the onset of symptoms?
Psychologic factors may be related to nocturnal enuresis.

Inquire about the quantity and timing of fluids consumed throughout 24 hours
Caffeinated beverages or late-night consumption of beverages can lead to nocturnal enuresis.

Is the pt taking diuretics or theophylline?
These medications can increase urinary frequency.

Have any of the family members had similar problems?
There is a positive family history of nocturnal enuresis in 50% of pts.

O **Perform physical exam**
Abdomen: Palpate for masses or distended bladder.
Urogenital: Inspect for any lesions or abnormal genitalia.
Back: Inspect for sacral dimpling or hair tufts.
Rectal: Assess sphincter tone, and check for hard stool in the vault.
Neuro:
 • Assess lower extremities for decreased motor strength or sensory changes.
 • Observe for abnormal gait.
 • Check for anal wink.

Consider the following labs and studies:
UA and urine culture
Renal and bladder ultrasound
Voiding cystourethrogram if UA or urine culture are positive
Lumbosacral x-rays if skin dimpling is present

Nocturnal enuresis is involuntary loss of urine that occurs at night (bedwetting) at the age of 5 years or greater
Primary enuresis: No history of having achieved nighttime urinary control
Secondary enuresis: History of having achieved prior nighttime urinary control (at least 6 months of no bedwetting) and now having involuntary loss of urine
Causes are multifactorial:
- Genetic component
- Functional bladder disorder: Small bladder capacity or bladder overactivity
- Maturational delay
- Vasopressin secretion: Decreased versus resistant antidiuretic hormone receptors
- Sleeping disorder: Obstructive sleep apnea, sleep arousal disorder
- Neurologic abnormality: Spina bifida, neurogenic bladder

 Recommend behavioral modifications
Bedwetting alarm: Moisture sensors on underwear, pajamas, and bed pads
Fluid restrictions: No fluids after dinner, no caffeinated beverages
Motivational therapy: Reward system of positive reinforcement
Bladder training: Attempts to delay urination during the day

Initiate pharmacotherapy: monotherapy or combination
Tricyclic antidepressants
Desmopressin
Long-acting anticholinergics
Oxybutynin

Refer
Urology referral is necessary if any urogenital abnormality is present.
Neurosurgery referral may be needed if neurologic anomaly is discovered.
Psychiatric evaluation is to be considered if the pt is currently undergoing psychological stressors.

S **Does the pt complain of a skin rash?**

Varicella begins as scanty papules usually on the face, spreads inferiorly to the trunk as papules, then transforms into vesicles and pustules that crust over.

Rubella usually has erythematous macules and papules that begin on the face and spread down to the trunk and extremities within 24 hours.

Measles rash presents with erythematous macules and papules that start on the face and neck, then spread centrifugally and inferiorly.

Coxsackie virus presents with multiple oral ulcer lesions with discrete, small, vesicular lesions of the hands and feet.

Erythema infectiosum has erythema and edema of the cheeks *("Slapped cheek")*.

Exanthema subitum can present as small, blanching macules or papules, with surrounding halos usually on the trunk and neck.

Is the rash pruritic or nonpruritic?

Many of the viral exanthems may be very pruritic, such as varicella.

Are there associated symptoms?

These viral rashes can present with fever, chills, malaise, coryza, sore throat, or arthralgias.

Ascertain if there was a recent upper respiratory infection (URI) before the rash.

Does the pt complain of gastrointestinal symptoms?

Viral exanthems can be associated with acute gastroenteritis, which may cause abdominal pain, nausea, vomiting, or diarrhea.

Any sick contacts with similar symptoms?

Most of the viruses are extremely contagious, and multiple cases may be seen from the same school, daycare, or family household.

Collect past medical history

Review pt immunization status and medications.

Pt may be at increased risk if immunodepressed or history of chronic disease.

O **Check vital signs**

Check for fever

Perform physical exam

HEENT: Perform a complete exam if there are URI symptoms.
- Check neck for nuchal rigidity for signs of meningitis.
- Examine for conjunctivitis.
- *Forchheimer's sign* is petechia on the soft palate, which are found in rubella and mononucleosis.
- *Koplik's spots* are clusters of tiny bluish-white papules with erythematous borders on the buccal mucosa in measles.

Heart: Auscultate for a rub that may indicate pericarditis.

Skin:
- Describe type, location, and appearance of the rash.
- Check for erythema, swelling, tenderness, or increased warmth.
- Look for breaks in skin, papules, macules, vesicles, blisters, or bullae.
- Examine the scalp for lesions.
- Lesion can have sharp borders or coalesce.

Musculoskeletal: Examine joints if involved.
Lymphatics: Check lymph nodes.
- Streaking redness may indicate lymphatic spread.

Consider the following labs and studies
CBC if systemic symptoms are present
Viral cultures
X-rays to rule out osteomyelitis or foreign bodies
Serum human herpes virus type 6 if suspect roseola infantum
Serum rubella antibody test
Serum parvovirus antibody if suspect erythema infectiosum
Serum Epstein-Barr virus antibody if suspect mononucleosis
Serum varicella virus antibody

Rash/Viral Exanthems
Causes:

- Varicella (chickenpox)	- Rubella (German measles)
- Measles	- Coxsackie virus (Hand, foot, and mouth disease)
- Mononucleosis	- Erythema infectiosum (Fifth disease)
- Enteroviral	- Roseola infantum (Exanthem subitum)

Provide supportive therapy
Antihistamines for pruritus
Topical corticosteroids for inflammation and pruritus
Oatmeal baths and calamine lotion for symptomatic relief
Antipyretics for fever defervescence
Oral or topical antibiotics for secondary bacterial infections

Prevention and education
Educate pt about skin care.
- Avoid scratching lesions to prevent secondary bacterial infection.
Discuss methods to reduce viral transmission.
- Quarantine pt if indicated.
- Instruct pt in proper hand-washing techniques and hygiene.
- Have pt avoid close contact if possible.
Immunize pt or family members with measles/mumps/rubella (MMR) vaccine or
varicella vaccine if indicated.

S **What symptoms is the pt experiencing with the respiratory infection?**
Pts may present with symptoms of rhinorrhea, sore throat, cough, fever, and
posttussive emesis.

Is the pt having trouble breathing?
Episodes of perioral cyanosis, nasal flaring, sternal retractions, and subcostal
retractions are all signs of respiratory distress.
Ingestion of a foreign body can cause respiratory distress.

Has the pt had any sick contacts?
Pts attending daycare or living with young siblings are prone to upper respiratory
infections (URIs).

Does the pt have a significant past medical history?
Infants and children with a history of prematurity, chronic heart disease, or chronic
lung disease are at risk of developing an apneic spell and severe disease.

Are all immunizations up to date?
Immunizations help protect from known causes of respiratory infections, such as
H. influenzae, S. pneumoniae, B. pertussis, and influenza virus.

O **Check vital signs**
Check for hypoxemia on pulse oximetry monitor.

Perform physical exam
General: Observe to see if the pt is alert or lethargic.
HEENT:
- Inspect oropharynx for clear or mucopurulent nasal discharge, blisters, petechia,
  ulcerations, enlarged tonsils, or enlarged uvula.

  ◆ *Do not examine the oropharynx in pts with epiglottitis who have copius drooling
    and are tripoding forward to breathe, because examination may further
    compromise the airway.*

- Palpate for submandibular or cervical lymph nodes.
- Listen for stridor in the neck and observe for supraclavicular retractions,
  suggesting airway compromise.
Chest:
- Look for intercostal retractions.
- Auscultate lung fields for rhonchi, crackles, wheezing, decreased breath sounds,
  or egophony.

Consider the following labs and studies:
CBC
Neck x-ray when stridor is heard
CXR
Respiratory syncytial virus (RSV) rapid antigen test

Respiratory Infection
Upper Respiratory Infection (URI):
- Croup   - Epiglottitis
- Laryngitis   - Pharyngitis
- Rhinitis   - Sinusitis
Lower Respiratory Infection (LRI):
- Bronchitis   - Bronchiolitis
- Croup   - Pneumonia

Most infections are caused by viral or bacterial agents
Parainfluenza virus is known for causing the laryngotracheobronchitis in croup, which leads to the characteristic "barking cough."
- "Steeple sign" is seen on anterior-posterior view of the neck x-ray.

Haemophilus influenzae is a bacteria known to cause epiglottitis, characterized by the forward-sitting, tripoding infant who is drooling.
- "Thumb sign" is seen on lateral neck x-ray.

Bordatella pertussis is a bacteria known to cause a characteristic staccato cough ending with a whoop ("whooping cough").

RSV, adenovirus, parainfluenza virus, and influenza virus are all known to cause bronchiolitis, inflammation of the bronchioles of the lungs.

URIs and LRIs can trigger reactive airway disease, causing hypersensitivity of airways and leading to constriction

Admit any pt with respiratory distress or airway compromise
Croup: Humidified oxygen, nebulized racemic epinephrine, systemic corticosteroids
Epiglottitis: Antibiotics
Bronchiolitis: Humidified oxygen, nebulized albuterol, nebulized racemic epinephrine
Pneumonia: Antibiotics

Treat symptoms of pts with less serious infections by using:
Bronchodilators for symptoms of wheezing
Cool mist from the shower for mild symptoms of croup
Oral antibiotics for bacterial pharyngitis, bronchitis, pneumonia, or sinusitis
Antipyretics for fever and myalgias
Dextromethorphan to help suppress the cough at night
Nasal decongestant for symptomatic improvement in rhinitis

S **What symptoms does the pt have suggesting a urinary tract infection (UTI)?**

Pts report frequency, hematuria, incontinence, urgency, nocturia, dysuria, foul-smelling urine, enuresis, or hesitancy.

Associated symptoms may include nausea, vomiting, and fever.

If there is pain, where is it located?

Pts can complain of burning on urination when a urethritis is present.

Lower back pain or flank pain suggests a kidney infection.

Has the pt had prior UTIs?

Diagnostic studies will depend on the age and gender of the pt and the number of UTIs.

Did the pt recently have any trauma or surgery?

Catheterization, circumcision, and abdominal or pelvic surgeries can predispose pts to UTIs.

Review family history

Vesicoureteral reflux does have familial predilection.

O **Check vital signs**

Check for signs of fever and ensure that the pt is hemodynamically stable.

Perform physical exam

Abdomen: Palpate to check for suprapubic tenderness, distended bladder, or palpable mass.

Back: Palpate for costovertebral angle tenderness.

Urogenital:
- Male pts should be checked to see if they are circumcised or not.
  - ◆ Check for phimosis.
  - ◆ Inspect for location of the urethral meatus, any lesions, or discharge.
- Female pts should have the urethral opening inspected for lesions and discharge.
  - ◆ If female is sexually active, a pelvic examination should be done to assess for cervical motion tenderness and adnexal or uterine mass.

Consider the following labs and studies:

In infants, urine specimen is obtained by suprapubic aspiration or bladder catheterization.

In older children, obtain urine specimen via bladder catheterization or midstream clean-catch technique if pt is capable.

UA suggestive of infection:

| - Bacteria | - Nitrite positive |
| - Blood | - Leukocyte esterase positive |

Send urine culture:
- If done via suprapubic aspiration, any bacterial growth suggests infection.
- If obtained by bladder catheterization, $> 10^4$ colonies suggests infection.
- If collected via midstream clean-catch, $> 10^5$ colonies suggests infection.

Collect gonorrhea/chlamydia cultures if history or physical exam indicates risk.

CBC, chemistry panel, blood cultures if pt looks toxic

UTI in the pediatric population
Predisposing factors:
- Constipation   - Local irritants: Bubble baths
- Renal abnormalities   - Uncircumcised male
- Sexual activity

Types:
- Lower UTI: Infection restricted to bladder (cystitis)
- Upper UTI: Infection involving kidney (pyelonephritis)

Two mechanisms include:
- Hematogenous spread and bacterial ascension

Etiologic agents:
- Most UTIs are caused by gram-negative bacteria:
  - *Escherichia coli*   - *Klebsiella*
  - *Proteus*
- Most common gram-positive bacteria involved:
  - *Staphylococcus saprophyticus*   - *Staphylococcus aureus*
  - *Enterococci*

P **Diagnostic workup requires an ultrasound to detect obstructive uropathy if:**
First UTI in a pt who is 2 years or younger, male or female
First UTI in a male regardless of age
Second UTI in female older than 5 years of age
Pt with pyelonephritis
Pt with poor response to antibiotics after 48 hours

Voiding cystourethrogram (VCUG) with contrast should be obtained to detect vesicoureteral reflux
VCUG is performed in the hospital after a second urine specimen is clean or after antibiotic therapy is completed.
If not scheduled promptly, pt continues on prophylactic dose of antibiotics.

Renal scan with technetium-labeled dimercaptosuccinic acid or glucoheptonate should be obtained to detect renal scarring
If pt has pyelonephritis or if VCUG revealed grade three or higher reflux

Treat lower UTIs with a 7-day course of antibiotics:
Trimethoprim-sulfamethoxazole
Cephalosporins
Nitrofurantoin

Treat upper UTIs with a 10- to 14-day course of antibiotics
Admit for IV antibiotics; switch to orals when pt has been afebrile for 48 hours.
Refer to Urology.

IV

Dermatology

S **What are the pt's symptoms?**
Acne can present as papules, pustules, nodules, comedones, or scarring.
Almost all teenagers are affected to some extent with acne.
In the elderly, sun-exposed areas of the face erupt with comedones called
   Favre-Racouchot syndrome.

Where is the acne location?
Acne commonly appears on the face, back, and chest.

What exacerbates or worsens the acne?
A high-fat diet or chocolate has *not* been shown to cause acne.
If the pt perceives that a food worsens acne, then have pt avoid that food.

Is the acne yearlong or seasonal?
Symptoms usually worsen in hot or humid climates.
Female pts often have acne erupt during times of menstruation.

What medication has the pt used and with what results?
Many pts want a quick fix, but treatment results may take months.
Certain medications, such as lithium, phenytoin, systemic corticosteroids, or
   progesterone-base contraception, can cause acne.

Does the pt have risk factors for acne?
Risk factors include male sex, adolescence, anabolic steroid abuse, pregnancy,
   contraceptive pills, contact skin irritants, oil-based cosmetics, or family history.
About one-half of pts with acne will have a family history of acne.

Is there a history of a virilization disorder?
Infantile acne can be seen as early as 3 to 6 months as a result of excessive androgens.
Up to 20% of neonates will have closed comedones.
Acne seen between ages 1 to 7 years should have a hyperandronergic workup.

O **Perform physical exam**
Skin: Examine for closed (whiteheads) or open (blackheads) comedones.
   • Comedones are usually dispersed over forehead, cheeks, nose, back, shoulders, or
     chest.
   • Check for papules, pustules, nodules, or cysts.
   • Pathologic findings can be seen, such as scarring, oily skin, thick skin,
     perifolliculitis, or sebaceous gland hypertrophy.
   • Scars can be described as ice pick, depressed, hypertrophic, or atrophic.
   • Look for telangiectasia, which may suggest rosacea.

A **Acne**
Categorize into three different types by its appearance:
- Comedonal
- Papular/Pustular
- Nodulocystic

Document severity:
- Mild to severe
- If no comedones are present, consider other causes such as folliculitis, dermatitis, chloracne, rosacea, pseudo-folliculitis barbae, and cosmetic or steroid-induced acne.

P **Treatment depends on the severity of the disease, location of the lesions, and pt's adherence with treatment options**
Recommend a healthy diet
Implement skin care
Advise pt to wash skin twice daily with mild or bacterial soap.
Avoid oily cosmetics.

Start pharmacotherapy
Antibacterial and keratolytic creams, gels, or solutions are first-line treatments.
Benzoyl peroxide works well for comedonal acne.
- Preparation in gel, soap, or lotion form can be used bid.

Salicylic acid
Naphthoic acid derivative (retinoid-like)
- Adapalene

Retinoic acid-derivative creams and gels for treatment of mild to moderate acne
- Tazarotene
- Tretinoin

Dicarboxylic acid antimicrobial cream, which is a keratinolytic, antibacterial, and anti-inflammatory treatment for inflammatory papules and pustules
- Azelaic acid

Antibiotics for colonization of *Propionibacterium acnes* in papular/pustular acne

- Tetracycline	- Minocycline
- Doxycycline	- Clindamycin
- Erythromycin	- Metronidazole
- Trimethoprim-sulfamethoxazole	

Isotretinoin (Accutane): For severe inflammatory acne that is unresponsive to conventional therapy (monthly CBC, LFT, and triglycerides checks needed)
Intralesional injection with corticosteroids
Estrogen/progestogen combination birth control pills

Caution should be used with female pts because some of the above agents can be teratogenic, especially isotretinoin.

Educate pt
Educate pts that treatment results are slow and can take up to 4 to 6 weeks.
Discuss contraception, sex, drug or alcohol use, or other health issues.
Stress reduction may be helpful.

S **Does the pt complain of an intermittent pruritic rash?**

Atopic dermatitis (AD) is an eczematous rash that can cause pruritus, erythema, papules, and pustules associated with dry skin.

Pruritus is the most common symptom associated with the rash.

AD can present as early as the first two months of life.

What exacerbates the pt's rash?

Foods, clothing, inhalants, medications, and skin products can exacerbate rash.

Frequent showers, baths, or washing with hot water can worsen the problem.

Pt can have AD associated with emotional stress, pregnancy, or menstruation.

Is the rash seasonal?

Improves in the summer and worsens in the winter when the pt's skin has a tendency to become xerotic.

Does the pt have a past medical history of associated diseases?

History of asthma, allergic rhinitis, or medication allergies can be present.

Also, endocrine disorders that cause dry skin, such as thyroid disease or diabetes, can be associated with AD.

Infections such as herpes, bacterial (streptococcus), or fungal infections can exacerbate AD.

Ascertain pt's family history

A family history of AD, asthma, or allergic rhinitis is common.

AD has a genetic predisposition.

O **Perform physical exam**

HEENT: Check for cataracts (seen in some pts).

Skin:

- Look for erythematous papules, plaques, pustules, or patches over flexor areas, side of neck, forehead, face, eyelids, wrist, and dorsa of the hand and foot (genital area can also be affected).
- Examine for associated scales, moist crusted erosions, skin swelling, or edematous surrounding rash.
- Scratching can cause excoriations and lichenification.
- Check hands, fingers, and feet for painful fissures.
- Look for hair loss over areas of scratching.
- Hypopigmented dermatographism can be expressed with rubbing of skin.
- Eyelids can be pigmented secondary to chronic rubbing.
- *Dennie-Morgan sign*: An infraorbital fold on the eyelid
- In darker-skinned pts, follicular papules are noticeable.
- Infants can have confluent edematous and erythematous vesicles with skin scaling, peeling, and fissures over the face, trunk, and extensor areas.
- Older children can have AD in flexor areas of arms (antecubital fossa) and legs (popliteal fossa) associated with papules, erosions, crusts, and lichenified lesions.
- Keratosis pilaris and ichthyosis vulgaris can be associated with AD.

Consider the following labs:

Check serum IgE, which can be elevated in 80% to 90% of pts with AD.

Skin bacterial/viral culture if primary or secondary infections are suspected

Atopic dermatitis is also known as eczema, atopic eczema, or IgE dermatitis

 Treatment goals are to provide immediate relief, place skin condition into remission, and reduce or prevent recurrences
Start pharmacotherapy
Oral or topical antihistamines for pruritus:
* Hydroxyzine
* Diphenhydramine
* Doxepin if severe pruritus
* Second-generation antihistamines listed in Allergic Rhinitis (p. 6)
Topical corticosteroids from low to high potency (avoid using high potency on face)
Immune-modulator macrolactam ascomycin derivative
* Pimecrolimus (Elidel)
Topical or oral antibiotic if secondary infection from scratching or rubbing
* *Staphylococcus aureus* can be associated with lesions.
Oral antiviral if herpes simplex is suspected
In severe cases, a short course of oral corticosteroids can be used.
Phototherapy with UVA-UVB or PUVA can be instituted.
Cyclosporine A has also been used, but it is associated with many side effects, and pt should be referred to a dermatologist for treatment.

Treat skin
Moist dressing to skin
Topical corticosteroids
Plastic occlusion can be used to increase absorption of corticosteroids into skin.
Hydrate skin with nonfragrant warm oil or oatmeal baths.
Topical antihistamines for pruritus

Educate pt
The number of baths per week should be reduced if possible.
Minimize soap usage.
Increase daily fluid intake.
Avoid irritants that may exacerbate symptoms.
Educate pt about proper application of steroid creams and discuss risks and benefits.
Use relaxation techniques and stress management if there are emotional triggers.
Provide reassurance.

What is the pt's description of the offending lesion?
Basal cell carcinoma (BCC) is a malignant tumor that causes local destruction of tissue.
Metastasis is very rare.

How long has the pt had the lesion?
Incidence of BCC is usually after the age of 40 years from repetitive sun exposure and
  lack of proper suncreen protection.

What is the shape, color, location, and size of the lesion?
BCC may start as a smooth, well-defined nodule.
Later stages may progress into a pigmented or colored lesion with telangiectasia.
Ulceration and crusting may also be seen in late stages.

Lesions are usually located in sun-exposed areas, most commonly on the nose.

Does the pt have risk factors?
Risk factors include fair skin, blond hair, blue eyes, and difficulty tanning.
Risk increases with number of years of ultraviolet sun exposure.
Exposure to ionizing radiation or arsenic is associated with BCC.
Pts with previous history of BCC have an increased likelihood of recurrence.

 Perform physical exam
Skin: Allow pt to disrobe so that the entire skin surface can be examined.
  - *Check **ABCDE** criteria for diagnosis of skin cancer* with good lighting and a hand
    lens:
    - ◆ *Asymmetry*: Compare one-half of the lesion to the other half.
    - ◆ *Border irregularity*: Look for border irregularity or unevenness.
    - ◆ *Color variegation*: Examine for more than one color (pigmented).
    - ◆ *Diameter*: Lesions larger than 6 mm can be highly suspicious.
    - ◆ *Elevation*: Check for lesions elevated above the skin surface.
  - Usually a single lesion but may have multiple lesions.
  - Check nasolabial folds, canthi, and ears.
  - Check for pearly or translucent papules or nodules (nodular).
  - Lesions can be crusted over ulcerations with rolled borders.
  - Lesion can mimic a scar (cicatricial).
  - Examine for pink or red thin plaques with telangiectasia (superficial).
  - Check for whitish patches with inconspicuous borders (sclerosing).

Consider the following procedure:
Shave or punch biopsy

 Basal Cell Carcinoma
Clinical types
  - Pigmented
  - Nodular
  - Cicatricial
  - Sclerosing
  - Superficial

P **Treatment goals are to remove BCC with clear margins, preserve normal function, and attempt to return normal appearance of resected site**

Implement nonsurgical treatment:
- Topical 5-fluorouracil ointment
- Imiquimod cream
- Photodynamic dye and visible light
- If the lesion is 2 mm or less, use the following methods to remove the lesion (only if it is not on the face because treatment may leave a scar).
  - Cryotherapy
  - Electrocautery and curettage

Perform surgical treatment:
- Facial BCC should be treated with excision and primary closure with skin flaps or graphs.
- Mohs' surgery should be performed if lesion is located in the nasolabial folds, canthi, or posterior ears.
- Excision should have clear 2- to 3-mm margins.

Educate pt

Reduce sun exposure.

If sun exposure is necessary, protect skin with clothing coverage or sunscreen.

Teach pt how to perform skin self-exam.

S **What is the pt's description of the bite or incident?**
It is important to obtain information about what or who bit the pt.
Ascertain the events surrounding the attack and where the bite is located.
Most bites are to the extremities.
Human bites can be accidental or are seen after fights, usually from punches to the
  mouth or teeth.

If bitten by an animal, was the animal domestic or wild?
Most animal bites are by domestic animals, usually dogs or cats.
Obtain vaccination history if the animal is a domestic pet.

Does the pt complain of fever or chills?
Infection risks are highest in cat and human bites.

Does the pt have a history of chronic disease?
Pts with chronic disease may have a higher risk for infections.

O **Check vital signs**
Check cardiovascular stability.

Perform physical exam
Skin: Check all skin areas involved.
  • Look for swelling, erythema, and broken skin.
  • If discharge is present, obtain a culture.
Musculoskeletal:
  • Examine tendons, bones, and joints located under or near bites to rule out
    tenosynovitis, fractures, or septic joint.
  • Check range of motion.
Lymphatics: Palpate for lymphadenopathy.

Consider the following labs and studies:
CBC if systemic symptoms or signs of infection
Bacterial cultures if indicated
X-rays to rule out fracture, osteomyelitis, or foreign body

A **Bites**
Human
  • Common organisms
      - Streptococci viridans   - *Staphylococcus epidermidis*
      - *Staphylococcus aureus*   - *Haemophilus influenzae*
      - *Eikenella corrodens*   - Anaerobic bacteria
Animals
  • Dogs
      - *Pasteurella multocida*   - *Staphylococcus aureus*
      - *Bacteroides* species   - *Fusobacterium* species
      - *Capnocytophaga canimorsus*
  • Cats
      - *Pasteurella multocida*   - *Staphylococcus aureus*
  • Wild animals (raccoons, bats, foxes, skunks, coyotes, squirrels)
      - Always consider rabies

Treatment
Admit for IV antibiotics if pt has systemic symptoms or an infection that has not responded to oral antibiotic treatment.
Place tetanus vaccine if indicated.

Treat human bites
Irrigate wound thoroughly with sterile saline and iodine.
Do not suture human bites, but allow closure by secondary intention.
Bandage wound with sterile gauze.
Splinting may be indicated if tendons or bones are involved.
Extremity injury should be elevated to reduce swelling.
Start antibiotic therapy:
- Amoxicillin-clavulanate (Augmentin)
- If pt has a penicillin allergy use:
  - Doxycycline in adults
  - Erythromycin in children
- Alternative antibiotics include:
  - Clindamycin and fluoroquinolone in adults
  - Clindamycin and trimethoprim-sulfamethoxazole in children
  - Daily IM ceftriaxone if pt noncompliant

Treat dog and cat bites
Treatment as per human bites

Do not suture if bite is on the hands, wrists, or feet, but allow closure by secondary intention.
Puncture wound should also be left open.
Primary closure of wound can be done if bite is less than 8 hours old.
Dogs should be quarantined for 10-day observation.
- If not possible, pt should be treated prophylactically for rabies.
Assess risk for rabies in dog bites and treat as stated below.

Treat wild animal bites
Treatment as per human bites
If at risk for rabies, place rabies immune globulin and human diploid cell rabies vaccine within 48 hours of the bite.

Implement prevention
Warn pt to always be aware of surroundings.
Domestic pets should have vaccinations and proper training.

S **Does the pt have a serious burn that needs admission?**

Serious burns are:
- Large area of first- and second-degree burns (> 20% of body surface area)
- First- or second-degree burns to hands, feet, groin, buttocks, face, or large joints
- Pts with third-degree burns (> 10% of body surface area)

These pts may need to be transported by ambulance to the ER.

What type of burn did the pt sustain?

First-degree burns are usually sustained by flash flames, scalding, or sunburns.

Second-degree burns are usually with hot liquids, solids, flash flames, electricity, or chemicals.

Third-degree burns are caused by the same items as second-degree burns.

Does the pt complain of pain, fever, or chills?

Pt can develop bacteremia and become septic.

How old is the pt?

Remember, children and elderly pts have thinner skin and burn easier.

O **Check vitals**

Confirm that pt is hemodynamically stable.

Perform physical exam

General: Estimate percentage of body surface area burned using rule of nines.

- Each area is estimated by 9% in adults (except genital region = 1%)
  - Head and neck (9%)   - Each arm (9%)
  - Torso (18%)/Back (18%)   - Each leg (18%)

- Palm rule: The palm is about 1% for quick estimations.

Skin: Check skin for burn type:
- First-degree burns appear superficial, dry, erythematous, and are painful initially.
  - Later these burns may peel and scar with discoloration.
- Second-degree burns extend into the dermis with pain, erythema, and moist blisters.
- Third-degree burns are full-skin thickness, dry, leathery, charred, and painless.
  - Third-degree burns usually have mixed colors from white to charred.

A **Burns**
Clinical types
- *First degree*: Involves superficial layer of the skin only
- *Second degree*: Involves extension into the dermis or partial thickness
- *Third degree*: Involves the entire skin depth into the subcutaneous layer or full thickness

P **Admit pt to hospital or special burn unit if burn is serious**
Stabilize pts with major burns for transport:
- Perform ABCs.
- IV fluids should be started to prevent shock until pt is transferred to emergency room.
- Remove burned clothing unless it is adherent to skin.
- Cover with sterile petroleum jelly or nonstick gauze bandage.
- Transfer pt to hospital.

Treat minor burns in the office
Place burn under cold water or cold compresses.
If second-degree burns present, do not break blisters.
Place moisturizer or aloe vera over very superficial burns.
Apply and prescribe topical antibiotics:
- Silver sulfadiazine (Silvadene)
- Mafenide (Sulfamylon) covers suspected *Pseudomonas*.
- Silver nitrate solution
- Bacitracin

Cover with sterile petroleum jelly or nonstick gauze bandage.
Provide pain management.
Monitor for signs of infection.
Update tetanus vaccine.

Implement prevention
Advise pt to have working smoke alarms in the home.
- Test them weekly.
- Replace batteries every 6 months.

Install plastic covers over electrical outlets.
Do not smoke in bed.
Parent or pt should check water temperature before using.
Set water heater to 120°F or less to prevent hot-water burns.
Keep children away from stove while cooking.
Turn handles of pots and pans toward the middle or the back of the stove.
Keep chemicals out of children's reach.
When handling chemicals, advise pt to wear protective gloves.

S **Does the pt complain of skin redness, swelling, or pain?**
Cellulitis is an expanding infection of the dermis and subcutaneous tissue.
Usually associated with skin pain, tenderness, and erythema.
Breaks in the skin can develop into more severe infection, such as osteomyelitis.

Is there associated fever, chills, or malaise?
More severe or regional cellulitis can develop into bacteremia or sepsis and cause fever,
chills, and malaise.

Was there a recent upper respiratory infection (URI)?
Facial cellulitis can rapidly develop after a pharyngitis or otitis media infection.

Is the infection located around the eye?
Periorbital cellulitis can develop into orbital cellulitis and cause proptosis or pain with
movement of the extraocular muscles.

How fast has the infection spread?
Necrotizing fasciitis, a medical emergency, spreads rapidly, usually with exaggerated
pain outside of erythema.

Does the pt have risk factors for cellulitis?
A history of trauma, recent surgery, diabetes, burns, IV drug use, or
immunocompromised states may increase risk for cellulitis.
Pts with venous or lymphatic insufficiency have a higher risk of developing cellulitis.

O **Check vital signs**
Check for hemodynamic stability.

Perform physical exam
HEENT: Perform a complete exam if complaint of URI, facial, head, or neck cellulitis is
present.
Skin:
- Check for erythema, swelling, tenderness, or increased warmth.
- Look for breaks in skin.
- Examine scalp for painful nodules.
- Borders can be sharp or ill-defined.
- Check for exquisite tenderness that extends outside the erythema.
- Look for streaking redness, indicating lymphatic spread.
- Outline border of erythema to assess improvement or worsening with follow-up
  visits.
Musculoskeletal: Examine tendons and joints proximal, distal, and under the cellulitis.
Lymphatics: Check lymph nodes.

Consider the following labs and studies:
CBC if systemic symptoms are present
Bacterial cultures if suspect bacteremia or sepsis
X-rays to rule out osteomyelitis or foreign bodies

Cellulitis
Common organisms:
- Group A streptococci   - *Staphylococcus aureus*
- Enterobacteriaceae   - *Pseudomonas*
- Anaerobic bacteria   - Fungi
- *Haemophilus influenzae* in facial cellulitis
- Non-group A β-hemolytic streptococci in recurrent cellulitis

Admit pts who have systemic symptoms or infection that has not responded to oral antibiotic treatment for IV antibiotics
Begin general measures
If limbs are involved, have pt elevate and immobilize limb.
Perform daily dressing changes.
Incision and drainage may be indicated if abscess formation is present.
Apply cool moist dressing to skin to give pain relief.

Start pharmacotherapy
Antibiotic or antifungal treatment depends on organisms.
Empiric treatment in uncomplicated pts should cover gram-positive bacteria.
- Penicillins
  - Penicillin V, amoxicillin-clavulanate, or dicloxacillin
- Cephalosporins
  - IM ceftriaxone daily if pt is noncompliant
- Macrolides
  - Erythromycin, azithromycin, or clarithromycin if penicillin-allergic pt
If *Pseudomonas* suspected, add an aminoglycoside.
Clindamycin should be added if anaerobes are suspected or if pt is diabetic with a break in the skin.
Cellulitis involving the orbits should be treated in an inpatient setting with IV antibiotics.
Start antipyretics and pain management, if needed.

Implement prevention
Educate pt about skin care.
Have pt monitor skin.
Provide safety education.

Does the pt complain of rash with associated flu symptoms?
Lyme disease (LD) begins with an erythematous rash followed by flu-like symptoms.
Symptoms can include fever, chills, headaches, myalgias, or arthralgias.
Many pts may be asymptomatic.

How does the pt describe the rash or lesion?
Erythema chronicum migrans skin lesion is classic for LD.

- Erythema chronicum migrans is an annular skin lesion that starts as an erythematous plaque for weeks and then spreads peripherally with central clearing.
This lesion leads to chronic inflammation of the skin over the extremities, which results in sclerosis and atrophy (chronic acrodermatitis chronicium atrophicum).

Has the pt been in areas where ticks are common?
LD is common worldwide in mostly forested areas.
In the United States, ticks are found in the Northeast, upper Midwest, coastal California, and Oregon.

Does the pt have any musculoskeletal symptoms?
Joints can have redness, increased warmth, or swelling.
Joint pain is usually migratory and can last for months after infection.

Has the pt experienced any cardiac or neurologic symptoms?
Cardiac symptoms may arise as a result of heart block or pericarditis.
Neurologic deficits, such as weakness, paralysis, or neuropathy, may indicate disseminated disease.
Facial palsies such as Bell's palsy are commonly seen.

Does the pt have any mental changes?
Pts can have memory loss, hallucinations, psychotic behavior, dementia, or depression.

Any visual or optic symptoms?
Ophthalmic manifestations can include optic neuritis, iritis, keratitis, or retinal vasculitis.

 Check vital signs
Check for cardiovascular stability.

Perform physical exam
General: Screen for abnormal behavior or mental changes.
HEENT:
- Check neck for nuchal rigidity or lymphadenopathy.
- Look for iritis, keratitis, retinal vasculitis, or optic neuritis on funduscopic exam.
Heart: Auscultate for abnormal heart sounds, such as bradycardia or rub.
Abdomen: Palpate for tenderness and liver enlargement.
Urogenital: Perform testicular exam for orchitis.
Musculoskeletal: Examine all large joints thoroughly.
- Look for swelling, pain, redness, and warmth.
Skin: Check for the classical erythema migrans and chronic acrodermatitis chronicium atrophicum.

Consider the following labs and studies:
ELISA for IgM/IgG *Borrelia burgdorferi* antibodies
Cerebrospinal fluid (CSF) or synovial culture for *Borrelia burgdorferi* if brain or joint
   infections
ECG if heart block suspected

A **Lyme disease is caused by the spirochete *Borrelia burgdorferi*, which is
transmitted by Ixodid ticks**
Stage 1: Erythema migrans with flu-like symptoms
Stage 2: Early disseminated disease with one or two organ systems involved
Stage 3: Chronic arthritis and neurologic syndromes

P **Admit pt if severe systemic symptoms
Start pharmacotherapy**
In adults, treat pts with doxycycline for 14 to 21 days.
In growing children, treat with amoxicillin for same amount of time.
If pt has severe symptoms with a normal CSF, treat for 28 days.
Corticosteroids can be used 5 to 7 days for inflammation.
If CSF is positive, pt will need one of the following medicines for 4 weeks IV:
   - Ceftriaxone   - Cefotaxime
   - Cefuroxime   - Penicillin G
Pregnant women should be treated with IV antibiotics (teratogenic tetracyclines should
   be avoided).

Implement prevention
Wear protective clothing that covers skin well when outdoors.
Insect or tick repellent should be used.
Check skin often if there is an area of exposure.
Remove tick immediately if bitten.
Bring tick for identification.
LYMErix is a three-dose vaccine that can be given for high-risk groups or populations
   in endemic areas.

S **What is the pt's description of the offending lesion?**
Symptoms are usually associated with a change in a pigmented lesion.
The lesion can change shape, color, size, or may crust and bleed.

Where is the lesion located?
Lesions are usually found in sun-exposed areas but can also be found on the feet, genitals, and legs.

What is the pt's risk for melanoma?

Assess risk factors by using MMRISK developed by The Brendan Society:

- <u>M</u>oles: Are there more than five atypical moles?
- <u>M</u>oles: Are there more than 50 common moles?
- <u>R</u>ed hair and freckling: Are these traits present?
- <u>I</u>nability to tan: Does the pt have difficulty tanning?
- <u>S</u>unburn: Has the pt been severely sunburned during preadolescent years?
- <u>K</u>indred: Is there a family history of melanoma?

Congenital giant/small nevus or dysplastic melanocytic nevus may predispose pts to developing melanoma.
Pts may be at risk for melanoma with one or more of the factors listed above.

O **Perform physical exam**
Skin: Allow pt to disrobe so that the entire skin surface can be examined.

- Check ABCDE criteria for diagnosis of skin cancer with good lighting and a hand lens:

  - *Asymmetry*: Compare one-half of the lesion to the other half.
  - *Border irregularity*: Look for border irregularity or unevenness (Wood's lamp can help define borders).
  - *Color variegation*: Examine for more than one color.
  - *Diameter*: Lesions larger than 6 mm have high suspicion.
  - *Elevation*: Check for lesions elevated above the skin surface.
- Check areas where melanoma is usually present:
  - Scalp
  - Back
  - Around mouth, rectum, and vulva
  - Medial knees and ankles in women
  - Toes and soles in darker-skinned pts

Lymphatics: Palpate regional lymph nodes for involvement.

Consider the following labs and studies:
Shave or punch biopsy for pathology
Epiluminescence microscopy
If *stage I or II* primary melanoma without palpable nodes, obtain:

      - CXR   - LFT
      - Lactate dehydrogenase
      - Lymphatic mapping with sentinel node procedure
        if thickness > 1.5 mm

If *stage III* primary melanoma with local or regional disease, obtain:
-   CBC   - LFT
-   CT scan of affected region   - LDH

If *stage IV*, obtain same as stage III plus:
-   CT scan of chest   - MRI of head
-   Bone scan   - GI series if gastrointestinal symptoms
                                                    present

A **Melanoma**
Clinical types depend on the time of the radial growth phase.
-   Superficial spreading
    -   Most common, with increased incidence in women
    -   Radial growth phase can be months to years.
-   Nodular
    -   High incidence in Japanese
    -   Radial growth phase can be 6 months or less.
-   Lentigo maligna
    -   Least common and not seen in pts with dark skin
    -   Radial growth phase can be years to decades; therefore, it is usually seen in much older individuals with years of sun exposure.
-   Desmoplastic
    -   Rare and usually lacks color
    -   Radial growth phase can be months to years.
-   Acral lentiginous
    -   Arise on the palms, soles, and nail beds
    -   Radial growth phase can be years.
-   Malignant melanoma of the mucosa
    -   Very rare
    -   Arises from the mucosa of the gastrointestinal, respiratory, and urogenital tracts
    -   Seen in blacks and East Indians

P **Treatment goal is early detection and removal of primary lesion before metastasis**
Remove lesion via surgical intervention
Total excisional biopsy can be done with narrow margins.
Complete surgical resection is indicated.
Sentinel lymph node procedure may be indicated.

Refer to Dermatology, Surgery, and Oncology in advanced disease
Educate pt
Reduce sun exposure.
Use skin protection with clothing coverage or sunscreen.
Teach pt how to perform skin self-exam.

S   **Does the pt complain of tiny flesh-colored papules?**
Molluscum are benign viral lesions that appear as small umbilicated papules.

How long has the pt had the lesions?
Incubation is about 2 weeks to 2 months, and lesions can persist up to 6 months.
Molluscum is usually self-limiting.

Where are the papules located?
Molluscum is usually located on the face, trunk, and extremities in children and on the
genitals in adults.

Are there symptoms associated with the lesions?
Lesions can be tender and itchy.

Does the pt have warts?
Verruca are painless benign viral lesions caused by the human papilloma virus (HPV).
Warts are described as hyperkeratotic papules or plaques with cleft surfaces or
vegetations.

Does the lesion bleed when scraped or cut?
Warts can bleed because the roots are supplied by capillary loops.

How long has the pt had the lesion(s)?
Verrucous lesions can persist for years.

Does the pt have risk factors for molluscum contagiosum or verruca?
Risk factors are close contact with an infected person, swimming pools, or
immunocompromised pt.

O   **Perform physical exam**
Skin:
- Molluscum
  - Examine skin for small flesh-colored papules with umbilicated centers.
  - Centers may have some erythema.
  - Papules can be grouped in one or two areas.
  - Look for nodules.
  - A white, creamy, keratotic plug can be expressed from the papules.
- Verruca
  - Examine skin for hyperkeratotic papules.
  - Look for filiform or cauliflower-like lesions.
  - Lesions can appear as well-defined papules and are usually painless.
  - Examine underneath hyperkeratotic tops of lesion for small red or brown
    spots from thrombosed capillaries (pathognomonic).
  - Colors of the lesions are usually flesh color, light brown, pink, or
    hypopigmented.

Consider the following labs and studies:
Molluscum is usually diagnosed clinically, but there are diagnostic tests:
- Smear of the keratotic plug with Giemsa stain usually shows inclusion of
  molluscum bodies.
- Biopsy shows intracytoplasmic inclusion bodies with hyperplastic and
  hypertrophied epidermis.

Verruca is also diagnosed clinically, but biopsy may reveal:
- Acanthosis, papillomatosis, koilocytosis, and hyperkeratosis

Molluscum contagiosum is a benign viral skin infection caused by the poxvirus
Verruca (warts) are caused by HPV
Clinical types:
- Common warts (verruca vulgaris)
- Plantar warts (verruca plantaris)
- Flat warts (verruca plana)
- Flat-top papules (epidermodysplasia verruciformis)

 Treat molluscum contagiosum if diagnosed
In healthy pts, molluscum will usually resolve spontaneously within 6 months.
Provide pain management if painful lesion.
Remove lesion with options listed as follows:
- Cryotherapy: Freeze for 10 to 15 seconds with liquid nitrogen.
- Imiquimod (Aldara) cream: Apply three times per week for 3 to 4 months.
- Removal with curettage
- If lesions are large nodules or unresponsive to therapies, laser surgery or eletrodesiccation can be used to remove lesions.

Treat verruca if diagnosed
Remove lesions with options listed as follows:
- Salicylic and lactic acid
- Imiquimod (Aldara) cream as above
- Cryotherapy: Freeze for 30 seconds with liquid nitrogen.
- Electrosurgery or surgical removal
- Hyperthermia: Plantar warts can be placed in hot water for 30 minutes three times per week.

Implement prevention
Avoid skin-to-skin contact until lesions resolve.
Educate pt about how to avoid possible autoinoculation.

S **Does the pt complain about skin lesions consistent with psoriasis?**
Lesions can be small, intermittent, eruptive inflammations or large, chronic, stable
  scaly plaques.

Where are the lesions located?
Psoriasis lesions are usually located on the elbow, knee, or scalp.

Is pruritus associated with the lesion?
Psoriasis can be extremely itchy and make the pt miserable.

Are there constitutional symptoms related to psoriasis?
Pt can complain of joint pain, fever, chills, fatigue, or weakness.
Pt may have a history of seronegative spondyloarthropathies, which are associated with
  psoriatic arthritis.

Does the pt have risk factors for psoriasis?
Risk factors include a family history of psoriasis, trauma, stress, or recent infections.
Streptococcal infection can exacerbate guttate psoriasis.

Is the pt taking medication that may precipitate psoriasis?
Medication such as:

- Alcohol	- ACE inhibitors
- β-blockers	- Morphine
- Lithium	- NSAIDs
- Antimalarial drugs	- Topical or oral corticosteroids
- Antibiotics such as tetracycline, penicillin, or sulfonamides	

O **Perform physical exam**
Skin:
  • Check for thickened symmetrical papules or plaques that have a salmon pink
    appearance with a dry silvery-white scale (discoid).
  • Scalp, eyebrows, intergluteal folds, extensors of arms, and knees are common
    sites for psoriasis.
  • Check nails for pitting or yellow-brown spots called oil spots (discoid).

  • Auspitz phenomenon: Small, pinpoint blood droplets can be seen when scales
    are peeled off.

  • *Koebner's phenomenon:* Psoriatic response 1 to 2 weeks after a skin injury
  • Look for diffuse, small papules concentrated over the trunk, usually in children
    (guttate).
  • Check palms and soles for small pustules (pustular).
  • If elderly pt, check flexor areas for moist, nonscaling lesions (flexural).
  • Check for generalized, exfoliating erythema over entire skin (erythroderma).
Musculoskeletal: Examine all large and small joints thoroughly.
  • Look for swelling, pain, redness, and warmth.

Consider the following study:
Biopsy: Can be done, but psoriasis is usually diagnosed clinically.

Psoriasis
Clinical types:
- Discoid or vulgaris (plaque)
- Guttate
- Pustular
- Inverse, flexural
- Erythroderma
- Ostraceous
- Psoriatic arthritis
  - *Distal*: Asymmetrical arthralgias of the distal interphalangeal joints
  - *Mutilating*: Bone erosion and osteolysis that result in ankylosis
  - *Axial*: Involvement of the sacroiliac, hip, and cervical spine
- Severe, unstable variants

Treatment depends on age, type, location, and extent of psoriasis
Referral to a dermatologist should be done initially to establish type and best treatment.
If pt has generalized or severe psoriasis, a dermatologist referral is indicated.

Implement general measures
Occlusive dressing with topical medications
Moist dressings can give symptomatic relief.
Oatmeal baths for pruritus
Arid weather may give relief.

Start topical medications
Salicylate acid
Calcipotriene (Dovonex)
Tazarotene
Coal tars
Corticosteroids: Low potency to high potency
Anthralin (Drithocreme): Can be used in conjunction with ultraviolet B (UVB)
  phototherapy.

Start oral medications for severe psoriasis
Methotrexate
Cyclosporine for severe psoriasis

Begin a trial intervention if severe
Interlesional corticosteroids
UVB phototherapy for generalized disease
Psoralen plus ultraviolet A (PUVA) photochemotherapy for generalized disease

Implement prevention
Avoid rubbing or scratching of skin.
Avoid drugs or medications that exacerbate psoriasis.

S **Does the pt complain of generalized itching, especially at night?**
Scabies are caused by a very contagious mite transmitted by close contact.

Nocturnal pruritus is common and may be severe.

Where does the pt complain of pruritus?
Pruritus coincides with hypersensitivity to the mite.
Burrow lesions are commonly found in these areas:
- Web spaces of fingers   - Hands
- Feet   - Wrists
- Genitals   - Waistline

Infants usually have lesions on the head and neck.

Does the pt complain of redness, vesicles, papules, or pustules?
Late manifestation of scabies includes vesicles and papules that can progress into
  erosions, excoriations, and pustules as a result of scratching.
Nodules can also be seen over buttocks, groin, axillae, or breasts.

Are there systemic symptoms such as fever or chills?
Staphylococcus aureus and Group A *streptococcus* infections can develop secondary to
  scratching.

Does the pt have risk factors for scabies?
Risk factors include recent skin-to-skin contact from sex, overcrowding, poverty, poor
  hygiene, and immunocompromised states.
Diffuse, crusting lesions may indicate an immunocompromised host.

O **Perform physical exam**
Skin: Examine the skin with a magnifying lens for burrows in areas stated above.
  • Burrows can be in a linear array, with a papule or vesicle at the end.
  • Look for mites at bottom of the burrows.
  • Check for erythema, papules, vesicles, pustules, and nodules.
  • Excoriations can be present from vigorous scratching.
  • In children, look for vesicular lesions of the palms and soles.

Consider the following studies:
Remove the mite with a 25-gauge needle and identify under the microscope.
Papules and vesicles can be scraped and mounted to check under the microscope for
  eggs, egg shells, feces, or mites.
Potassium hydroxide mount of scrapings can be used for the same finding described
  above.
Burrow ink test: Ink is place over affected skin and wiped with alcohol.
  • Remaining ink identifies burrows

Scabies
Cause
- The contagious mite *Sarcoptes scabiei*, var. hominis

Treat pt and all close contacts
Start pharmacotherapy
- Permethrin (Elimite) 5% cream
  - First-line therapy
  - Apply from head to soles of feet at night and wash off in the morning (avoid eyes, nose, and mouth).
  - One or two applications should suffice.
- Lindane (Kwell, Scabene) 1% lotion, shampoo, or cream
  - Apply the same as permethrin.
  - Contraindicated in seizure disorders or malnourished children
- Crotamiton (Eurax) 10% cream
  - Apply the same as permethrin, but apply two nights consecutively because it is less potent.
- Precipitated sulfur 6% in petroleum
  - Pts are usually nonadherent to this treatment because of odor and messiness.
  - Safe in infants and children
- Ivermectin plus one of the above creams in HIV-positive pts
- Topical or oral antihistamines or corticosteroids can be used if itching is severe.
Educate pt
- Teach about infection and prevention of spread.
- Advise pt to wash all clothing and linens.

What is the pt's description of the offending lesion?

Actinic keratosis (AK) is described as a discrete, rough, dry, or scaly lesion in a sun-exposed area.

Squamous cell carcinoma (SCC) can be described as a well-demarcated, scaly, erythematous plaque to a friable nodule or papule with hyperkeratosis or erosions.

The lesions can change shape, color, size, or may crust and bleed.

Where is the lesion located?

Usually in sun-exposed areas

How long has pt had the lesion?

Incidence of SCC is usually after age 55 years secondary to sun exposure and lack of proper suncreen protection.

In Australia and New Zealand, SCC can be seen as early as 20 to 30 years of age.

Does the pt have risk factors?

Risk factors include fair skin, blond hair, blue eyes, and difficulty tanning.

Risk increases with number of years of ultraviolet sun exposure.

Exposure to ionizing radiation or arsenic is associated with SCC.

Pts who work outdoors or who are immunocompromised have increased risk.

Is there a history of previous AK or SCC?

Pts with a previous history of AK or SCC have an increased likelihood of recurrence.

Perform physical exam

Skin: Allow pt to disrobe so that the entire skin surface can be examined.

- Check ABCDE criteria for diagnosis of skin cancer with good lighting and a hand lens:

  - ◆ *Asymmetry*: Compare one-half of the lesion to the other half.
  - ◆ *Border irregularity*: Look for border irregularity or unevenness.
  - ◆ *Color variegation*: Examine for more than one color.
  - ◆ *Diameter*: Lesions larger than 6 mm have high suspicion.
  - ◆ *Elevation*: Check for lesions elevated above the skin surface.
- Check sun-exposed areas:
  - - Scalp
  - - Cheeks
  - - Ears
  - - Neck
  - - Forehead and temples
  - - Nose
  - - Vermilion border of lower lip
  - - Extremities
- Examine skin for scaly, erythematous macules, or papules with central ulcerations (SCC).
  - ◆ Look for telangiectasia.
- Check for single or multiple rough, dry, or hyperkeratotic (scaly) skin lesions in sun-exposed areas (AK).
  - ◆ Hyperkeratotic areas are better felt with fingertips than visualized.
- Look for large brown and black variegated lesions with verrucous surface spreading laterally (spreading pigmented AK [SPAK]).

Consider the following study:

Skin biopsy

Squamous Cell Cancer
Caused by ultraviolet light and human papilloma virus

Actinic Keratosis
Clinical subtype
* SPAK

 Treatment consists of removal of lesions
Treat SCC if diagnosed
Electrodesiccation and curettage for small lesions
Lesions > 4 mm thickness will need excisional removal.
Lesions beyond the dermis will need resection and possible radiation or chemotherapy.
Specialized Mohs' surgery to obtain clear margins can be performed.
Metastatic SCC will need systemic chemotherapy and referral to an oncologist.

Treat AK if diagnosed
Cryotherapy with liquid nitrogen
5-Fluorouracil cream twice daily for 2 to 4 weeks
Retinoid creams
Trichloroacetic acid facial peel
Erbium or carbon dioxide laser surgery
Acitretin and isotretinoin (retinoid) oral treatment

Implement prevention
Advise pt to use sunscreen when in the sun.
Educate pt of symptoms, signs, and self-monitoring for skin cancer.
Avoid sun exposure during high UV times or days.
Wear protective clothing and hats.

S **What is the pt's description of the skin condition?**
Generally, tinea is described as being annular with well-demarcated erythematous
  borders and central clearing.
Papules, vesicles, and pustules may be seen near the border.
Lesions can be scaly or macerated.

Where is the lesion located?
The lesions are usually in moist, humid parts of the body, such as the axillae, feet,
  groin, or scalp.

How long has the pt had the lesion?
Infection can last for months to years.

Does the rash or lesion itch?
Pruritus is usually what brings the pt into the office.

Has the lesion increased in size over time?
Scratching may cause spreading and secondary lichenification.

Does the pt have risk factors for a fungal infection?
Risk factors may include:

- Use of public showers   - Poor hygiene
- Work with animals   - Children in school or daycare
- Chronic topical steroid use   - Immunocompromised pt
- Contact with an animal or person with a tinea infection
- Exposure to warm climates or being overclothed during hot, humid times

O **Perform physical exam**
Skin: Examine skin carefully.
- Capitis
  - Check scalp for round, scaly areas with black dots from broken hair or alopecia.
  - Look for kerions, which are exudative, pustular areas from chronic infection.
- Corporis/Facialis
  - Check face, truck, and extremities for annular, erythematous plaques with
    central clearing and well-demarcated borders.
  - Examine for papules or vesicles at the borders.
- Cruris
  - Check groin area for lesions similar to corporis.
- Pedis
  - Examine the feet for scaling, vesicles, and maceration.
- Manuum
  - Examine for erythema and scaling of the hands.
- Incognito
  - Check for neck and facial lesions with well-defined erythema.
- Barbae
  - Look for pustular folliculitis in the beard or mustache area.
- Versicolor
  - Check for multiple painless lesions from white to brown, usually over chest,
    shoulders, back, and face.

Consider the following labs or studies:
LFT if use of oral antifungals
KOH test under microscopy usually shows spores and hyphae.
Fungal culture of scrapings
Wood's lamp test can diagnose *Microsporum* species.

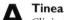 **Tinea**
Clinical types:

- Pedis (feet)	- Manuum (hands)
- Cruris (groin)	- Corporis (trunk, face, extremities)
- Facialis (face)	- Incognito (face, neck)
- Capitis (scalp)	- Barbae (beard area)

- Versicolor (can be seen over all skin areas)

Causes:

- Dermatophytes
  - *Trichophyton* species
  - *Epidermophyton* species
  - *Microsporum* species
  - *Pityrosporum* ovale (versicolor only)

P **Resolution may be spontaneous in 6 months in healthy pts without treatment**
Start topical antifungals

- Miconazole	- Clotrimazole
- Ketoconazole	- Econazole
- Naftifine	- Oxiconazole
- Sulconazole	- Terbinafine
- Tolnaftate	- Ciclopirox olamine

- Selenium sulfide shampoo for versicolor
- Clotrimazole-betamethasone (Lotrisone), a combination topical antifungal and corticosteroid, may be used initially if pt has marked inflammation.

Start oral antifungals if topical fails

- Griseofulvin	- Itraconazole
- Terbinafine	- Fluconazole

Use antihistamines to relieve pruritus
Implement general measures
Perform good hygiene.
Wash all clothing, linens, and towels.
Treat household or family members.
Wear open-toed shoes or sandals.
Antiperspirants should be used in moist areas of the body.
Pt can also use drying powders.
Change socks regularly.

S **What is the pt's description of the offending rash?**
Urticaria is a sudden itchy rash with single or many raised macules with red halos.
Also described as wheals or hives
Urticaria may occur anywhere on the body.

How long has the pt had the rash?
Rash usually spontaneously resolves rapidly in hours without any residual lesion.
Chronic urticaria can last more than 30 days.
Rash usually recurs intermittently.

What exacerbates the rash?
Rash may appear with stimuli such as stress, exercise, pressure, cold, heat, or sunlight.

Has the pt been ill?
Bacterial, viral, fungal, and parasitic agents have all been implicated as causes of
urticaria.
Helicobacter pylori infection seems to play a role in urticaria.

Does the pt complain of swelling of the lips, tongue, or throat?
Angioedema and generalized anaphylaxis can be associated and may be fatal.
Difficulty breathing with urticaria may indicate anaphylaxis.

Is there a past medical history or family history of related illnesses?
Atopic dermatitis, asthma, and allergic rhinitis may be associated with urticaria.

Do triggers cause the urticaria?
Review any new exposures to foods, drugs, plants, skin products, or chemicals that
might cause an allergic reaction.

 Check vital signs
Check airway and breathing.

Perform physical exam
General: Observe for facial swelling.
HEENT: Perform a complete exam to check for signs of angioedema.
Chest: Auscultate lung fields for decreased aeration or wheezing.
Skin:
  • Check for raised erythematous plaques with central pallor.

  • Scratch pt's skin to induce a raised rash (dermatographism).

Consider the following labs and studies:
CBC if evidence of infection
Stool ova and parasites if suspect parasitic infection
Serum eosinophil count
Skin biopsy in chronic cases only
ANA, ESR, and TSH if systemic diseases are suspected
Ice cube test if suspect cold-induced urticaria
Methacholine skin test if suspect cholinergic or exercise-induced urticaria
Solar exposure for heat-induced urticaria
Pressure application to skin to rule out pressure-induced urticaria

Urticaria
Causes

- IgE-mediated
- Complement-mediated
- Anti-FcεRI autoantibody-mediated
- Physical stimuli
- Idiopathic

P **Stop offending agent if determined**
Start pharmacotherapy
Antihistamines can give symptomatic relief.

- First generation causes sedation and is available over the counter:
  - Hydroxyzine
  - Diphenhydramine
- Second generation has less sedation:
  - Loratadine (Claritin)
  - Cetirizine (Zyrtec)
  - Desloratadine (Clarinex)
  - Fexofenadine (Allegra)

Tricyclic antidepressant

- Doxepin (Sinequan)

Oral corticosteroids for pts who are difficult to treat

- Prednisone taper can be given.

If infection is detected, treat appropriately.

Implement general measures
Apply cool, moist compresses to area.

V

Orthopedic Conditions

S **What sports will the pt participate in during the year?**
Clearance may be sport specific.

Are there any medical problems that may not allow pt to participate?
Ask about current medical problems at time of physical

Review pt's PMH:
Include a thorough cardiac history:

- Is there a family history of premature or sudden death?
- Any specific cardiac problems with pt or relatives?
- Does the pt have a history of cardiac murmur?

Review any hospitalizations.

Obtain FMH
See Adult History & Physical (p. 2).

Review SH
Include history of alcohol, tobacco, or drug use.
List all of the pt's medications or supplements.
Ask about nutrition, diets, weight gain or loss, hydration, and body image.
Inquire about heat-related illness.

Review of systems should include the following questions:
Neurologic:
- Does the pt have any history of sustaining head trauma or concussion?
- Any loss of consciousness or seizures?
- Any history of headaches?
- Ascertain if there has been any numbness, tingling, or paralysis of limbs.
- Has the pt sustained a "stinger" or pinched nerve?
Ophthalmologic:
- Does the pt require corrective lenses?
- Has the pt ever sustained trauma to the eyes?
Pulmonary:
- Does the pt have a history of asthma, wheezing, dyspnea with activities, or other pulmonary problems?
- Any allergies?
Cardiovascular:
- Has the pt ever had chest pain, syncope, or palpitations?
- Inquire about a history of hypertension, hypercholesterolemia, or obesity.
- Any recent viral illness that may indicate cardiomyopathy?
- Is the pt reporting excessive fatigue with activities?
Musculoskeletal:
- Any history of sprains, strains, fractures, tendonitis, dislocations, or subluxations?
- Does the pt require any orthopedic devices or braces?
Skin:
- Any skin infections or lesions?

O **Check vital signs**
Perform physical exam
General: Document any abnormalities (e.g., Marfan's syndrome).
HEENT:
- Examine visual acuity and pupils.
- Check mouth for loose or missing teeth, signs of an eating disorder, or chewing tobacco use.
- Examine tympanic membranes for perforations.
- Listen for carotid bruits and measure jugular venous distention.

Chest: Auscultate for crackles, wheezes, or other abnormal breath sounds.
Heart:
- Listen for a murmur and its location.
  - ◆ Timing: Murmurs can be systolic, diastolic, or holosystolic.
- Auscultate for clicks, gallops, trills, S_3 or S_4.
- A displaced point of maximal impulse indicates enlargement.

Abdomen: Palpate for hepatosplenomegaly, abdominal masses, or hernias.
Extremities:
- Check pulses in upper and lower extremities.
- Observe for cyanosis, clubbing, or edema.

Musculoskeletal: Assess the range of motion of all joints.
- Check muscular symmetry.
- Refer to specific joint topics for a complete exam of joint in question.

Neurologic: Perform full exam.
Skin: Look for any lesions.

Labs or studies are not indicated unless a specific problem is suspected; however, some practitioners obtain an ECG in all pts
If the ECG is abnormal, an echocardiogram is indicated.

A **Sports Medicine Screening Exam**

P **Treatment plan is to educate pt on safety and maintain healthiness during the different sporting activities**
Educate pt
Emphasize specific sport safety, protection, and prevention.
Discuss proper hydration and nutrition.
Discuss appropriate stretching and conditioning.
Review anticipatory guidance for injuries or specific medical problems.
Counsel on supplements, anabolic steroids, drugs, and alcohol.

Asthmatic pts should have an inhaler at all games or practices, and the trainer, teacher, or coach should have access to the inhaler in case of an emergency.

S

What are the pt's complaints?
Document symptoms related to the ankle/foot pain.

Does the pt have a history of trauma or ankle/foot problems?
If trauma, obtain a detailed description of the incident.
Inversion sprains are the most common injury to the ankle, usually from sports involving jumping or frequent change of direction.
Common foot problems are ingrown toenails, corns, bunions, hammer toes, midfoot sprains, heel spurs, or plantar fasciitis.

Where is the pain located?
Location is key to diagnosis.
Document if anterior (dorsal), posterior (plantar), lateral, or medial.
The pain may be of muscle, bone, ligament, vascular, or neurologic origin.

Ask about the duration and severity of the pain
The quality of the pain can be sharp, dull, achy, or numbing.

Ask what makes the pain better or worse?
Document treatments or medications that have made the pain better.

Is there morning stiffness?
Osteoarthritis starts with morning stiffness and improves with activity.

Any neurologic or radicular symptoms?
- Numbness   - Tingling   - Bowel/bladder incontinence
- Paralysis   - Weakness   - Balance or coordination difficulty

Review pt's activities, work duties, and hobbies
Does the pt have a history of medical problems?
Review pt's past medical problems and injuries, including a history of osteoarthritis, gout, pseudogout, rheumatoid arthritis, or fractures.
Constitutional symptoms may indicate malignancy.
A history of osteopenia or osteoporosis can increase pt's risk for injury or fracture.

Review pt's medications
Medications, illicit drugs, steroids, or alcohol may increase pt's risk for injuries.

O

Check vital signs
Fever may indicate septic joint.

Perform physical exam
Ankle/Foot:
- Check for swelling, crepitus, erythema, or ecchymosis.
- Palpate for pain, effusion, or increased warmth.
- Palpate for point tenderness for specific anatomic injury.
- Examine for muscular symmetry.
- Assess range of motion.
- Assess stance and gait.
- Perform neurovascular exam.
- Specific ankle test:
  - *Single-heel rise test*: Pt raises the heel, placing weight on ball of foot to assess Achille's tendon.
  - *Anterior drawer test*: Assess the anterior fibular ligament, by grabbing heel with one hand and pulling anteriorly, while the other hand provides stability to the distal tibia.

♦ *Inversion stress test:* To assess the calcaneofibular ligament, use the same method as the anterior drawer test, except apply inversion to the heel instead of pulling anteriorly.

Consider the following labs and studies:
X-rays of the ankle or foot if indicated
CBC if infection is suspected
CT scan or MRI if indicated
Bone scan if suspect osteomyelitis, malignancy, or occult fracture
Electromyography to rule out peripheral neuropathy or radiculopathy

Ankle/Foot pain
Common ankle etiologies
      - Ankle sprains   - Fractures   - Infection
      - Osteoarthritis   - Specific tendon injuries (e.g., Achilles, peroneal)
Common foot etiologies
      - Metatarsalgia   - Morton's neuroma   - Plantar fasciitis
      - Corns   - Hammer-toes   - Trigger toes
      - Fractures   - Infection (e.g., tenia pedis, septic joint)

P **Treat specific cause of pain**
Infected joints or bursitis will need to be aspirated and the pt placed on antibiotics.

Start pharmacotherapy for pain and inflammation
NSAIDs unless contraindicated
A short course of narcotics may be used if the pt is in severe pain.
If pt is having muscle spasms, a short course of muscle relaxants can be used.
Trigger point injection with corticosteroids may be used.

Implement RICE therapy (Rest, Ice, Compression, and Elevation)

Start general measures
Modified activity and work should be implemented.
Bracing may be indicated.
Promote weight loss and healthy diet.
Educate pt on proper safety, protection, stretching, and exercise.

Prescribe physical therapy when indicated
Cold and heat packs can be used.
Ultrasound for deep heat
Transcutaneous electrical stimulation and traction can be used.

Refer to a specialist:
If pt does not improve after 4 to 6 weeks

S **What are the pt's complaints?**
Document symptoms related to the back pain.

Does the pt have a history of trauma or back problems?
If trauma, obtain a detailed description of the incident.
Low-back injuries are a major cause of disability.

Where is the pain located?
Location is key to diagnosis.
Document if cervical, thoracic, lumbar, or sacral area of pain.
The pain may be from muscle, bone, ligament, vascular, or neurologic origin.

Ask about the duration and severity of the pain
The quality of the pain can be sharp, dull, achy, or numbing.

What makes the pain better or worse?
Document treatments or medications that have made the pain better.

Is there morning stiffness?
Osteoarthritis starts with morning stiffness and improves with activity.
Rheumatoid arthritis pain is worsened with activity.

Any neurologic or radicular symptoms?
    - Numbness   - Tingling   - Bowel/bladder incontinence
    - Paralysis   - Weakness   - Balance or coordination difficulty

Review pt's activities, work duties, and hobbies
Does the pt have a history of medical problems?
Review pt's past medical problems and injuries.
Constitutional symptoms may indicate malignancy.
A history of osteopenia or osteoporosis can increase risk for injury or fracture.

Review pt's medications
Medications, illicit drugs, steroids, or alcohol may increase risk for injuries.

O **Check vital signs**
Fever may indicate infection or malignancy.

Perform physical exam
If suspect a systemic problem, perform a complete physical exam.
General: Observe pt's posture, pain, distress, and movements.
Musculoskeletal:
  • Observe the unclothed back for asymmetry.
  • Palpate the back muscles and spine.
  • Evaluate gait and stance.
  • Perform range-of-motion exam of the back.
  • Test pt's mobility by assessing ability to stand, sit, and lie down.
Neuro:
  • Perform a complete neurologic exam, including deep tendon reflexes.
  • Perform straight-leg test to rule out sciatica or herniated disc.

Consider the following labs and radiographic studies:
Plain x-ray of the thoracic, lumbar, and sacral regions if indicated
CT or MRI if indicated
Bone scan if osteomyelitis, malignancy, or occult fracture is suspected
Electromyography to rule out peripheral neuropathy or radiculopathy

CBC if infection is suspected
PSA if history of prostate cancer or if it is suspected
ESR and CRP if inflammatory process is suspected
RF if signs and symptoms are consistent with rheumatoid arthritis

 Back Pain
Etiologies:

- Strains	- Osteoarthritis	- Acute disc herniation
- Spinal stenosis	- Malignancy	- Ankylosing spondylitis
- Fractures	- Infection	- Spondylolisthesis
- Cauda equina	- Referred pain from an internal organ	

 Treat specific cause of pain
Start pharmacotherapy for pain and inflammation
NSAIDs unless contraindicated
A short course of narcotics may be used if pt is in severe pain.
If pt is having muscle spasms, a short course of muscle relaxants can be used.
Trigger point injection with corticosteroids may be used.

Start general measures
Modified activity and work should be implemented if no neurologic signs.
Have pt avoid heavy lifting, pulling, or pushing.
If radiculopathy, prescribe a short 2- to 3-day bed rest in supine position.
Bracing or corsets may be indicated in compression fractures caused by osteoporosis.
Incorporate exercises that strengthen musculature.
Promote weight loss and healthy diet.

Educate pt about proper ergonomics, safety, protection, and posture to prevent reinjury in the future.

Prescribe physical therapy when indicated
Cold and heat packs can be used.
Ultrasound for deep heat
Transcutaneous electrical stimulation and traction can be used.

Refer to a specialist
If pt does not improve after 4 to 6 weeks
Referral to chiropractic services for spinal manipulation can be used.
Treat any psychological problem that may inhibit recovery.

S **What are the pt's complaints?**
Document symptoms related to the elbow pain.

Does the pt have a history of trauma or elbow problems?
If trauma, obtain a detailed description of the incident.
Most injuries to elbow are secondary to overuse.
Fractures of the elbow can commonly injure the ulnar nerve because of its location in the cubital tunnel.

Where is the pain located?
Location is key to diagnosis.
Document if anterior, posterior, lateral, or medial.
The pain may be from muscle, bone, ligament, vascular, or neurologic origin.

Ask about the duration and severity of the pain
The quality of the pain can be sharp, dull, achy, or numbing.

What makes the pain better or worse?
Document treatments or medications that had made the pain better.

Is there morning stiffness?
Osteoarthritis starts with morning stiffness and improves with activity.

Any neurologic or radicular symptoms?
- Numbness   - Tingling   - Bowel/bladder incontinence
- Paralysis   - Weakness   - Balance or coordination difficulty

Review pt's activities, work duties, and hobbies
Does the pt have a history of medical problems?
Review pt's past medical problems and injuries, including a history of osteoarthritis, gout, pseudogout, rheumatoid arthritis, or fractures.
Constitutional symptoms may indicate malignancy.
A history of osteopenia or osteoporosis can increase risk for injury or fracture.

Review pt's medications
Medications, illicit drugs, steroids, or alcohol may increase risk for injuries.

 Check vital signs
Fever may indicate septic joint or bursitis.

Perform physical exam
Elbow:
- Check for swelling, nodules, erythema, or ecchymosis.
- Palpate for pain, effusion, or increased warmth.
- Palpate for point tenderness for specific anatomic injury with the elbow flexed at 70 degrees.
    ◆ Palpate the olecranon, bursa, medial, and lateral epicondyles.
- Examine for muscular symmetry between both elbows.
- Assess range of motion.
    ◆ Perform extension, flexion, supination, and pronation.

Consider the following labs and studies:
Plain x-ray of the elbow if indicated
CT or MRI if indicated
Bone scan if osteomyelitis, malignancy, or occult fracture is suspected
Electromyography to rule out peripheral neuropathy or radiculopathy

CBC if infection is suspected
ESR and CRP if inflammatory process is suspected
Arthrocentesis may be indicated to rule out inflammation or infection process.

A **Elbow pain**
Common etiologies:

- Fractures (e.g., supracondylar)   - Infection
- Little leaguer's elbow   - Gout
- Olecranon bursitis   - Osteoarthritis
- Medial (golfer's elbow)/Lateral (tennis elbow) epicondylitis
- Radial head subluxation (nursemaid's elbow)

P **Treat specific cause of pain**
Radial head subluxation requires reduction by supination of the forearm while flexing the elbow to 90 degrees with pressure over the radial head until back in position.
Infected joints or bursitis will need to be aspirated and the pt placed on antibiotics.

Start pharmacotherapy for pain and inflammation: NSAIDs unless contraindicated
A short course of narcotics may be used if the pt is in severe pain.
If the pt is having muscle spasms, a short course of muscle relaxants can be used.
Trigger point injection with corticosteroids may be used.

Implement RICE therapy (Rest, Ice, Compression, and Elevation)

Start general measures
Modified activity and work should be implemented.
No lifting, pulling, or pushing heavy items if indicated.
Bracing may be indicated (e.g., tennis elbow band can be used in epicondylitis).
Educate pt on proper safety, protection, stretching, and exercise.

Prescribe physical therapy when indicated
Cold and heat packs can be used.
Ultrasound for deep heat
Transcutaneous electrical stimulation and traction can be used.

Refer to a specialist
If pt does not improve after 4 to 6 weeks

S **What are the pt's complaints?**
Document symptoms related to the knee pain.

Does the pt have a history of trauma or knee problems?
If trauma, obtain a detailed description of the incident.

Where is the pain located?
Document if anterior, posterior, lateral, or medial.

Ask about the duration and severity of the pain
The quality of the pain can be sharp, dull, achy, or numbing.

Does the knee give way, pop, or lock?
Popping suggests ligament injury, and locking suggests a meniscal tear.
"Giving way" may indicate ligament rupture or patellar dislocation.

Does the pt complain of swelling of the knee?
Rapid effusion may indicate a tibial plateau fracture or ACL tear.
Gradual effusion can be seen with meniscal tear or ligament injury.
Meniscal injuries can produce recurrent swelling after activity.

Is there morning stiffness?
Osteoarthritis starts with morning stiffness and improves with activity.

Review pt's activities, work duties, and hobbies
Does the pt have a history of medical problems?
Review pt's past medical problems and injuries, including a history of osteoarthritis,
gout, pseudogout, rheumatoid arthritis, or fractures.
A history of osteopenia or osteoporosis can increase risk for injury or fracture.

 Check vital signs
Fever may indicate septic joint or bursitis.

Perform physical exam
Knee
- Check for swelling, erythema, ecchymosis, effusion, or increased warmth.
- Palpate for point tenderness for specific anatomic injury.
- Examine for muscular symmetry and range of motion between both knees.
- Palpate patellar tracking.
  - Perform patellar apprehension test by subluxing the patella laterally.

Anterior drawer test or Lachman test can examine the ACL
Anterior drawer test: Pt supine with knee flexed 90°, foot mildly externally rotated, sit
on foot and wrap hands around lower leg over tibial tubercle, and pull anteriorly to
check for laxity.
Lachman test: Pt supine with knee flexed 30°, hold the distal femur stable with one
hand, grab proximal tibia with other hand, and pull tibia anteriorly to check for laxity.

Posterior cruciate ligament can be tested with the posterior drawer test
This is done by the same method as the anterior drawer test except the proximal tibia is
pushed posterior for laxity.

Examine the collateral ligaments
With pt supine, flex knee 30°, stabilize distal tibia with one hand, and with the other
hand, grab ankle and move it laterally and medially to check for laxity or pain.

Examine the menisci

Check for tenderness at the joint lines.

Perform the *McMurray test*:

- With pt supine, cup the anterior knee with your hand with the thumb on the lateral joint line and fingers over medial joint line; flex knee fully, place other hand over distal tibia from the medial side, and rotate tibia internally while applying valgus stress to medial joint line and extending the leg outward to test the lateral meniscus. (Apply varus stress to test medial meniscus.)

Perform an exam of the joints proximal and distal to the knee
Consider the following labs and studies:

Three-view x-rays of the knee	MRI if indicated
CBC if septic joint is suspected	ESR and CRP if inflammatory
RF if suspect rheumatoid arthritis	
Weight bearing x-ray of knee for osteoarthritis	
Arthrocentesis if inflammatory or septic joint is suspected	

 ### Knee Pain, differential by age of the pt

Pediatric pts:

- Osgood-Schlatter   - Osteochondritis dissecans   - Patellar subluxation
- Patellar tendonitis   - Slipped capital femoral epiphysis with referred pain

Adult pts:

- Medial plica syndrome   - Patellofemoral syndrome   - Pes anserine bursitis
- Trauma (fractures, sprain, strains, contusion, etc.)
- Septic joint   - Inflammatory arthritis such as rheumatoid or Reiter's syndrome

Elderly pts:

- Gout   - Osteoarthritis   - Pseudogout   - Popliteal cyst

 ### Treat specific cause of pain

See Osteoarthritis (p. 52) for treatment

Infected joints or bursitis will need to be aspirated and the pt placed on antibiotics.

Start pharmacotherapy for pain and inflammation

NSAIDs unless contraindicated

A short course of narcotics may be used if the pt is in severe pain.

Trigger point injection with corticosteroids may be used.

Implement RICE therapy (Rest, Ice, Compression, and Elevation)

Start general measures

Modified activity and work should be implemented.

Bracing may be indicated.

Incorporate exercises that strengthen musculature.

Promote weight loss and healthy diet.

Prescribe physical therapy when indicated
Refer to a specialist if pt does not improve after 4 to 6 weeks

S **What are the pt's complaints?**
Document symptoms related to the neck pain.

Does the pt have a history of trauma or neck problems?
If trauma, obtain a detailed description of the incident.
Whiplash injury is a common problem seen after car accidents.

Where is the pain located?
Location is key to diagnosis.
Document if anterior or posterior.
The pain may be from muscle, bone, ligament, vascular, or neurologic origin.

Ask about the duration and severity of the pain
The quality of the pain can be sharp, dull, achy, or numbing.

What makes the pain better or worse?
Document treatments or medications that have made the pain better.

Is there morning stiffness?
Osteoarthritis starts with morning stiffness and improves with activity.

Any neurologic or radicular symptoms?
      - Numbness   - Tingling   - Bowel/bladder incontinence
      - Paralysis   - Weakness   - Balance or coordination difficulty

Review pt's activities, work duties, and hobbies
Does the pt have a history of medical problems?
Review pt's past medical problems and injuries.
Constitutional symptoms may indicate malignancy.
A history of osteopenia or osteoporosis can increase risk for injury or fracture.

Review pt's medications
Medications, illicit drugs, steroids, or alcohol may increase risk for injuries.

O **Check vital signs**
Fever may indicate infection or malignancy.

Perform physical exam
General: Observe pt's posture, pain distress, and movements.
HEENT:
  • Check for jugular venous distention, bruits, masses, lymphadenopathy, dental exam, and oropharyngeal exam.
  • Examine eyes for eyelid drooping or pupillary abnormalities.
Musculoskeletal:
  • Observe the neck for symmetry.
  • Palpate muscles and spine.
  • Check for muscle atrophy, hypertrophy, or fasciculations.
  • Perform range-of-motion exam of the neck and extremities.
  • Evaluate gait and stance.
Neuro: Perform a complete neurologic exam, including deep tendon reflexes.
  • Examine the motor, sensory, and reflexes of C5, C6, and C8 nerve roots.

Specific neck exams that may indicate cervical compression
Arm abduction test: Pain resolves with placement of their hand on top of their head.
Axial compression test: Pain is felt with downward axial pressure while neck is in neutral position and relief with upward traction.

Lhermitte's sign: Electric-like pain shoots down arms with the neck fully flexed.
Spurling's test: Pain is felt with extension of the neck and rotation to the affected side.

Consider the following labs and studies:
Cervical x-rays if indicated
CT scan or MRI if indicated
Discography to view the disc
CBC if infection is suspected
Electromyography and nerve conduction to rule out peripheral neuropathy or
  radiculopathy

 Neck Pain
Etiologies:

- Muscular sprains/strains	- Ligament injuries	- Osseous
- Neurologic	- Cutaneous	- Inflammation
- Malignancy	- Infection	- Cardiac
- Degenerative disease	- Trauma	

- Referred pain from visceral organs
- Compression of neural structures (usually C5, C6, and C7 nerve
  compression by disc protrusion or osteophyte)

P **Treat specific cause of pain**
Start pharmacotherapy for pain and inflammation
NSAIDs unless contraindicated
A short course of narcotics may be used if the pt is in severe pain.
If pt is having muscle spasms, a short course of muscle relaxants can be used.
Trigger point injection with corticosteroids may be used.

Start general measures
Modified activity and work should be implemented if no neurologic symptoms.

If radiculopathy, prescribe a short 2- to 3-day bed rest in supine position.

A cervical collar or cervical traction device may be helpful.
Incorporate exercises that strengthen musculature.
Educate pt of proper ergonomics, safety, protection, and posture to prevent reinjury in
  the future.

Prescribe physical therapy when indicated
Refer to a specialist
If pt does not improve after 6 to 8 weeks
Referral to chiropractic services for cervical manipulation can be used.
Treat any psychological problem that may inhibit recovery.

S **What are the pt's complaints?**
Document symptoms related to the shoulder pain.

Does the pt have a history of trauma or shoulder problems?
If trauma, obtain a detailed description of the incident.
Shoulder dislocation is a common cause of pain with trauma.

What is the pain's location, duration, and severity?
Document if anterior, posterior, or lateral.
The pain may be from muscle, bone, ligament, vascular, or neurologic origin.
The quality of the pain can be sharp, dull, achy, or numbing.

What makes the pain better or worse?
Document treatments or medications that have made the pain better.

Any neurologic or radicular symptoms?

- Numbness	- Tingling	- Bowel/Bladder incontinence
- Paralysis	- Weakness	- Balance or coordination difficulty

Review pt's activities, work duties, and hobbies
Does the past have a history of medical problems?
Review pt's past medical problems and injuries.
Constitutional symptoms may indicate malignancy.
A history of osteopenia or osteoporosis can increase risk for injury or fracture.

Review pt's medications
Medications, illicit drugs, steroids, or alcohol may increase risk for injuries.

O **Check vital signs**
Fever may indicate septic joint or bursitis.

Perform physical exam
Shoulder:
- Check for swelling, erythema, or ecchymosis.
- Palpate for pain, effusion, or increased warmth.
- Palpate for point tenderness for specific anatomic injury.
  - Palpate the acromioclavicular (AC) joint, acromion, anterior glenohumeral (GH) joint, biceps tendon, coracoid process, scapula, and sternoclavicular joints.
- Examine for muscular symmetry between both shoulders.
- Assess range of motion with active and passive movements.
- Check the scapula for winging.

Examine the rotator cuff by testing the teres minor, infra-/supraspinatus, and subscapularis muscles
Test supraspinatus by having the pt extend arms out in front 90 degrees with thumbs pointing down, and have pt elevate arm over shoulders against resistance.
Test infraspinatus and teres minor by having pt place arm by the side with 90-degree elbow flexion, and apply resistance against external rotation.
Test subscapularis by having the pt place the dorsum of the hand on the lumbar area, and ask the pt to passively lift the hand off the back.

Perform specific provocative tests that may indicate the diagnosis
Perform the *Apley scratch test* (indicates rotator cuff injury): To test internal rotation and abduction, have the pt touch the opposite scapula overhand and underhand.

Perform the *Drop-arm test* (indicates rotator cuff tear): With arm adducted 90 degrees, have pt slowly lower arm to waistline.

Perform the *Apprehension test* (indicates anterior GH instability): With arm abducted and flexed 90 degrees, externally rotate the arm and apply anterior pressure over the biceps.

Check for the *Sulcus sign* (indicates inferior GH instability): Check for indentation lateral to the acromion when you pull a neutral arm downward.

Check for the *Clunk sign* (indicates a labral disorder): With pt supine, rotate arm while applying resistance with extension and forward flexion.

Perform the *Cross-arm test* (indicates AC joint arthritis): With the pt's arm elevated to 90 degrees, have pt adduct arm across body.

Perform the *Yergason test* (indicates biceps tendon problem): With the arm flexed 90 degrees, grab the wrist and have the pt supinate and flex against resistance.

Neck and elbow should be examined

Perform the *Spurling's test* (indicates cervical nerve problem): With cervical spine in extension and head toward injured shoulder, push down on the top of the head to reproduce radiating pain downward toward the elbow.

Consider the following labs and studies:
X-rays to rule out fracture or osteoarthritis
MRI or CT scan if indicated
CBC if septic joint is suspected
ESR or CRP if inflammation
Arthrocentesis if inflammatory or septic joint is suspected

A **Shoulder pain**
Common etiologies:

- Arthritis	- Sprains/strains	- Tendonitis
- Fracture	- Rotator cuff tears	- Frozen shoulder
- Impingement syndrome	- Dislocation	- Separation

P **Treat specific cause of pain**
Infected joints or bursitis will need to be aspirated and the pt placed on antibiotics.

Start pharmacotherapy for pain and inflammation
NSAIDs unless contraindicated
A short course of narcotics may be used if the pt is in severe pain.
If pt is having muscle spasms, a short course of muscle relaxants can be used.
Trigger point injection with corticosteroids may be used.

Start general measures
Modified activity and work should be implemented.
No lifting, pulling, or pushing heavy items if indicated.
Educate pt on proper safety, protection, stretching, and exercise.

Prescribe physical therapy when indicated
Refer to a specialist:
If pt does not improve after 4 to 6 weeks

S **What are the pt's complaints?**
Document symptoms related to the wrist/hand pain.

Does the pt have a history of trauma or wrist/hand problems?
If trauma, obtain a detailed description of the incident.
Wrist and hand fractures are common.

Where is the pain located?
Location is key to diagnosis.
Document if anterior (palmar), posterior (dorsum), lateral, or medial.
The pain may be from muscle, bone, ligament, vascular, or neurologic origin.

Ask about the duration and severity of the pain
The quality of the pain can be sharp, dull, achy, or numbing.

What makes the pain better or worse?
Document treatments or medications that have made the pain better.

Is there morning stiffness?
Osteoarthritis starts with morning stiffness and improves with activity.
Rheumatoid arthritis usually worsens with activity.

Any neurologic or radicular symptoms?
     - Numbness   - Tingling
     - Paralysis   - Weakness

Review pt's activities, work duties, and hobbies
Repetitive injuries to the hand or wrist can present with the above symptoms.

Does the past have a history of medical problems?
Review pt's past medical problems and injuries, including a history of osteoarthritis,
   gout, pseudogout, rheumatoid arthritis, or fractures.
A history of osteopenia or osteoporosis can increase risk for injury or fracture.

Review pt's medications
Medications, illicit drugs, steroids, or alcohol may increase risk for injuries.

O **Check vital signs**
Fever may indicate infection.

Perform physical exam
Wrist/hand: Check for swelling, bony enlargement, erythema, or ecchymosis.
   • Perform specific test for carpal tunnel:
      ◆ *Tinnel's sign*: Test for pain by tapping over the median nerve of palmar side of
        the wrist.
      ◆ *Phalen's sign*: Test for reproducible symptoms with maximum flexion at the
        wrists
   • If suspect osteoarthritis, check distal interphalangeal joints for *Heberden's nodes*
     and proximal interphalangeal joints for *Bouchard's nodes*.
   • If suspect rheumatoid arthritis, check for bilateral deformity of the
     metacarpophalangeal joints with ulnar deviation.
   • Palpate for pain, effusion, or increased warmth.
   • Palpate for point tenderness for specific anatomic injuries.
      ◆ Palpate the anatomic snuffbox to rule out a scaphoid fracture.
   • Examine for muscular symmetry between both wrists/hands.

◆ Check symmetry of thenar and hypothenar muscles to rule out medial or ulnar nerve compression, respectively.
● Assess range of motion.
  ◆ Check flexion and extension.
  ◆ For the thumb, also include adduction, abduction, and opposition.
● Check tendons for contractures or thickening.
● Examine the sensation of distribution of the medial, radial, and ulnar nerves.

 Wrist/Hand Pain
Common etiologies:

- Carpal tunnel	- Dislocations	- Fractures
- Gamekeeper's thumb	- Ganglion cyst	- Mallet finger
- Osteoarthritis	- Sprains/strains	- Tenosynovitis
- Dupuytren's contractures	- Rheumatoid arthritis	- Trigger finger
- Infections (e.g., septic joint, felon, paronychia)		

P **Treat specific cause of pain**
Infected joints or bursitis will need to be aspirated and the pt placed on antibiotics.
See Osteoarthritis (p. 52) for treatment.

Start pharmacotherapy for pain and inflammation
NSAIDs unless contraindicated
A short course of narcotics may be used if the pt is in severe pain.
Trigger point injection with corticosteroids may be used.

Implement RICE therapy (Rest, Ice, Compression, and Elevation)

Start general measures
Modified activity and work should be implemented.
No lifting, pulling, or pushing heavy items if indicated.
Splinting, casting, or bracing to provide immobilization may be necessary.
Educate pt on proper safety, protection, stretching, and exercise.

Prescribe physical therapy when indicated
Cold and heat packs can be used.
Ultrasound for deep heat
Transcutaneous electrical stimulation and traction can be used.

Refer to a specialist:
If pt does not improve after 4 to 6 weeks

VI

Psychiatry/Psychosocial Issues

S   **What is the quantity and frequency of the pt's alcohol use?**
Remember that a standard drink contains 14 g of pure alcohol:
- 12 ounces of beer or wine cooler
- 8–9 ounces of malt liquor
- 5 ounces of table wine
- 3–4 ounces of fortified wine
- 2–3 ounces of cordial, liqueur, or aperitif
- 1.5 ounces of brandy
- 1.5 ounces of 80-proof spirits

Rule of thumb for "too much" is 7 drinks per week or > 3 drinks per occasion for women or elderly, and 14 drinks per week or > 4 drinks per occasion for males.

Ask the CAGE questions:
Has the pt ever felt that he or she should Cut down?
Have people Annoyed the pt by criticizing his or her drinking?
Does the pt feel Guilty about his or her drinking?
Has the pt ever had an Eye-opener?
- The pt may be dependent if he or she answered "yes" to three or four questions.
- The pt may have alcohol-related problems if he or she answered "yes" to one or two questions.
- The pt may still have a problem even though "no" was answered to all questions.

Does the pt have any symptoms of withdrawal?
Withdrawal symptoms include difficulty sleeping, tremors, seizures, nervousness, anxiety, or hallucinations.

Has alcohol use caused problems with the law, health, social life, work, or relationships?
Drinking while pregnant can be deleterious to the baby and mother.
Absenteeism, tardiness, frequent job changes, or decreased work productivity may be secondary to a drinking problem.
Substance abuse is involved in more than half of motor vehicle deaths and domestic violence cases.
Pts with depression or anxiety may be self-treating with alcohol.
Sexual dysfunction such as erectile dysfunction may be related to alcohol abuse.

Does the pt have a medical problem caused by alcohol?
A myriad of medical and psychological conditions can be associated with alcohol dependency.

Does the pt have a family history of alcohol or drug addiction?
There appears to be a genetic disposition for alcoholism.

O   **Check vital signs**
Check for tachycardia or labile blood pressures, which may suggest withdrawal.

Perform physical exam
General: Check for gross defects, such as tremor or speech impediments.
HEENT:
- Check eyes for nystagmus, dilated pupils, or icterus.
- Note alcohol odor on breath.

Chest: Perform complete exam.
Heart: Check for tachycardia or displaced point of maximum impulse, which may indicate an enlarged heart.
Abdomen:
- Check for abdominal pain.
- Examine for an enlarged liver, ascites, or masses.

Skin: Look for spider angioma, caput medusae, palmar erythema, and jaundice.

Consider the following labs and studies:
Serum alcohol level
Gamma-glutamyl transpeptidase and LFT
Mean corpuscular volume for folate and vitamin B_{12} deficiency
Carbohydrate-deficient transferrin can indicate prolonged malnutrition.
Random urine drug screen if other drug use suspected

 Alcoholism

 Assess pt's desire to quit
Pt has to be ready to quit.
Advise pt of your concerns.

Implement a plan with the pt
Be nonjudgmental, empathetic, and nonconfrontational.
Depending on readiness of the pt, advise to cut down or stop all together.
Allow pt to be involved in planning and setting feasible goals.
Have close follow-up and congratulate pt if following treatment plan.

Refer to support groups
Alcoholics Anonymous
Narcotics Anonymous
National Drug and Alcohol Treatment Referral Routing Service phone number
- 1-800-662-HELP

Substance Abuse Facility Treatment Locator website
- http://findtreatment.samhsa.gov

Refer to psychologist or psychiatrist
If co-existing mental disorders are involved

Admit for detoxification to an inpatient or outpatient setting if necessary

S **Does the pt complain of anxiety or panic attacks?**
Anxiety is characterized by excessive worrying about several events or activities in the pt's life for more than 6 months.

Panic attack is characterized by recurrent, unexpected attacks of intense fear that begin abruptly and reach a peak within 10 minutes.

Are there multiple complaints of vague symptoms?
Review multiple symptoms that must satisfy criteria listed in the assessment.

Is there a pt history or family history of psychologic disorders?
There is a genetic predisposition for anxiety and panic attacks.

Does the pt have a history of medical problems or drug abuse?
The attacks or anxiety cannot be caused by a medical or substance abuse problem.

Review current or past medications or supplements

O **Check vital signs**
Perform physical exam if symptoms suggest organic cause
Chest: Perform a complete pulmonary exam.
Heart: Check for abnormal heart sounds or murmurs (e.g., mitral valve prolapse).

Perform mental status exam
General appearance and behavior: Check grooming, hygiene, attitude, psychomotor assessment, and eye contact.
Affect: Blunted, flat, or labile
Mood: Check for depressed mood.
Thought process: Assess speech and thoughts.
Thought content: Ask about suicide, hallucinations, delusions, and depersonalization.
Cognitive evaluation: Assess level of consciousness, orientation, attention and concentration, memory, basic knowledge, calculations, abstraction, insight, and judgment.

Consider the following labs:
CBC if signs of infection
Chemistry panel
RUDS if drug abuse
RPR to rule out syphilis if suspected
Serum alcohol level
TSH if suspect thyroid disease

A **Generalized Anxiety Disorder/Panic Attack diagnosis has to meet the Diagnostic and Statistical Manual of Mental Disorder (DSM-IV) criteria**
Diagnostic criteria for general anxiety disorder
Excessive anxiety or worrying is present most days during at least a 6-month period about several events or activities in the pt's life.
Pt is unable to control anxiety.
The pt has at least three of the following symptoms:

- Easy fatigability	- Difficulty concentrating
- Irritability	- Muscle tension
- Sleep disturbance	- Restlessness

Anxiety cannot be about anticipation of a panic attack.
The anxiety causes deficits in the pt's daily functions.

The symptoms cannot be caused by a general medical condition or substance-induced mood disorder.

The symptoms cannot be caused by a psychotic disorder.

Diagnostic criteria for panic attacks

Unexpected recurrent panic attacks and intense fear with four of the following symptoms that begin abruptly and reach a peak within 10 minutes:

- Chest pain or discomfort   - Sweating
- Paresthesias   - Feeling of choking
- Fear of dying   - Chills or hot flashes
- Derealization or depersonalization   - Dizzy or lightheadedness
- Nausea or abdominal discomfort   - Trembling or shaking
- Palpitations or increased heart rate   - Shortness of breath or sensation
- Fear of losing control or going crazy

At least one of the attacks is followed by 1 month of one of the following:

- A persistent concern about having another attack
- Worrying about what might happen during the attack
- A change in behavior because of the attacks

The attacks cannot be caused by a medical or substance abuse problem.

The attacks cannot be caused by another psychologic problem.

P Institute nonpharmacologic treatment

Relaxation techniques or meditation

Stress reduction

Biofeedback

Start psychotherapy

Cognitive behavior therapy alone or in combination with pharmacotherapy

Start pharmacotherapy if anxiety or attacks result in functional impairment

Benzodiazepines:

- Alprazolam (Xanax)   - Chlordiazepoxide (Librium)
- Clonazepam (Klonopin)   - Clorazepate (Tranxene)
- Diazepam (Valium)   - Lorazepam (Ativan)
- Oxazepam (Serax)

SSRIs, tricyclic antidepressants, and other anxiolytics, such as buspirone (Buspar) or β-blockers, can be used (see list in Depression p. 186).

Educate pt and family about the disease
Provide support groups, which can be beneficial
Referral may be indicated in pts with comorbidities or complicated cases

S **What are the pt's symptoms?**
Bipolar pts can have changes in mood that range from elation to depression.
Mania is usually described as a period of one week with symptoms of abnormally
  elevated, expansive, or irritable mood, with three or more of the following symptoms:

- Inflated self-esteem or grandiosity   - Decreased need for sleep
- Pressured speech   - Flight of ideas or racing thoughts
- Very distractible   - Increase in pleasurable activity
- Psychomotor agitation or increased goal-directed activity

See Depression (p. 186) for specific symptoms.
In children, there can be symptoms of hyperactivity or temper-tantrums.
Affects men and women equally, and onset is usually in late teens to the mid-thirties.

How are the symptoms of mania, hypomania, and depression related to each other?
Obtain history of how the moods are related and if the pt is cycling.

Is there evidence that pt engages in high-risk behaviors?
Pts may experience impaired judgment or act on impulses.

Are the symptoms triggered by psychosocial stressors?
Mood changes are usually triggered by stressors.

Is there a pt history or family history of psychologic disorders?
There is a genetic predisposition for bipolar disorder.

Does the pt have a history of medical problems or drug abuse?
The symptoms cannot be caused by a medical or substance abuse problem.

Review current or past medications or supplements

O **Perform a complete physical exam if symptoms suggest an organic cause**
Perform mental status exam
General appearance and behavior: Check grooming, hygiene, attitude, psychomotor
  assessment, and eye contact.
Affect: Blunted, flat, or labile
Mood: Check for depressed mood
Thought process: Assess speech and thoughts
Thought content: Ask about suicide, hallucinations, delusions, and depersonalization.
Cognitive evaluation: Assess level of consciousness, orientation, attention and
  concentration, memory, basic knowledge, calculations, abstraction, insight, and
  judgment.

Consider the following labs:
CBC if signs of infection
Chemistry panel
RUDS if drug abuse
RPR to rule out syphilis if suspected
Serum alcohol level
TSH if suspect thyroid disease
UA if taking lithium
Serum levels of mood stabilizers

A **Bipolar I and II diagnosis have to meet the Diagnostic and Statistical Manual of Mental Disorder (DSM-IV) criteria**
Diagnostic criteria for Bipolar I
One or more Manic or Mixed episodes
With a history of one or more major depressive episodes, but not required for diagnosis
Manic or Mixed episodes cannot be caused by a medical problem, substance abuse, medications, or treatment for depression.
Cannot be caused by psychotic disorder
Diagnostic criteria for Bipolar II
One or more major depressive episodes and at least one hypomanic episode
Manic or Mixed episodes cannot be caused by a medical problem, substance abuse, medications, or treatment for depression.
Cannot be caused by psychotic disorder

P **Admit pt if in acute manic or depressive state**
Educate pt and family about bipolar disorder and anticipatory guidance
Implement general measures
Avoid alcohol or illicit substance use.
Firearms should not be kept in the home.
Sexually transmitted infection education and testing when indicated
Anticipatory guidance regarding financial matters
Support groups can be beneficial.
Regular office visits and telephone contacts with the pt and family are crucial.

Start pharmacotherapy
Mood stabilizers (Remember to monitor levels and labs.)
  • Lithium
  • Valproic acid (Depakote)
  • Carbamazepine (Tegretol)
Antidepressants in conjunction with mood stabilizers
  • SSRIs (see Depression p. 186)
  • Bupropion (Wellbutrin)
Benzodiazepines can be used for sedation and sleep regulations.
Antipsychotics can be used in mania with psychosis and psychotic depression.

Referral to psychiatrist is usually indicated

S **What is the pt's complaint?**
Take a complete and descriptive history of events and persons involved.
If possible, take separate histories from the caregiver and child.
Include all of the people who care for the pt in the histories.
Is the history inconsistent with injuries?
Injury sustained may not be age appropriate or correlate with physical exam.
Suspicion should arise if caregiver delayed seeking medical care for the child.
Caregiver may admit to inflicting injury on the child.
Ask about pt's past medical history or review chart?
Child may have a history of injuries over time that are suspicious.
Review past medical history and medications.
Does the child have a medical condition that may mimic child abuse?
Hematologic: Hemophilia, thrombocytopenia, Henoch-Schönlein purpura, and von Willebrand's disease
Dermatologic: Phytophotodermatitis, Mongolian spots, vascular malformations, and subcutaneous fat necrosis
Infectious: Bullous impetigo, staphylococcal scaled skin syndrome, and petechia or purpura from bacterial or viral infections
Congenital metabolic disorders: Osteogenesis imperfecta, Ehlers-Danlos syndrome, and rickets
Insensitivity-to-pain disorders
Accidental trauma: Toddler's fracture and stress fracture
Does the pt have risk factors for child abuse?
Delay in development
Children with complicated medical conditions
Unwanted or abandoned children
Very fussy or difficult children, who may present with colic or hyperactivity
Parent or caregiver who is under tremendous stress
Parent or caregiver with unrealistic goals or developmental expectations of the child

O **Check vital signs**
Check height, weight, and body mass index.
Perform physical exam
General:
  • Document any abnormalities.
  • Look for evidence of neglect or failure to thrive.
HEENT:
  • Carefully examine the scalp.
  • Examine the eyes for retinal hemorrhages.
  • Check mouth for loose teeth or trauma.
  • Examine tympanic membranes for perforations.
Chest: Look for abnormal respirations.
Heart: Perform a complete heart exam.
Abdomen: Examine abdomen and genital area for abuse.
Extremities: Check pulses in upper and lower extremities.

Musculoskeletal:
- Assess all joints for range of motion.
- Refer to specific joint topic for a complete exam of joint in question.
- Palpate for bony tenderness.

Neurologic: Perform a complete exam, especially in suspected "shaken-baby" syndrome.

Skin:
- Look for any lesions, such as bruises, in areas not normally seen:

  | - Buttocks | - Ears | - Frenulum |
  | - Thighs | - Torso | - Neck |

- Examine for burns that look circumferential from immersion.
- Check for bite marks.
- Any lesion with well-demarcated shapes (e.g., belt buckle, cigarette, fist)
- Inspect for hand marks from grabbing.
- Look for lesions with multiple healing stages.
- Palpate all body surfaces.
- Photograph each lesion.

Consider the following labs and studies:

CBC if signs or symptoms of anemia or infection
PT/PTT if bruising or bleeding disorder suspected
X-rays of specific sites in questions
Skeletal survey if the child is less than 2 years old
CT scan of the head if suspected neurologic injury
Bone scan can be obtained in occult fractures.

A   **Child Abuse**

P   **Treat pt's injuries appropriately**
Inform parents or caregiver about concern of abuse and steps required by law that must be taken to protect the child

Notify Child Protective Services in all cases where abuse is suspected.
Documentation is crucial and should be done carefully.

Place child

Depending on findings, a medical decision needs to be made whether to hospitalize the pt, place in protective custody, or send home with parent.

S **Does the pt complain of sadness or depression?**

An easy acronym (***SIG E CAPS***) can be used to recognize depression in pts:

- Sleep disturbance
- Interest or pleasure lost
- Guilty feeling of worthlessness
- Energy reduction or fatigue

- Concentration or attention deficit
- Appetite/weight changes
- Psychomotor disturbances
- Suicidal ideation or plan

Assess pt's suicide risk and evaluate for warning signs

Pts who are very agitated, having hallucinations or delusions, or experiencing labile moods can be at risk for suicide.

Be aware of subtle comments or signs of impending suicide or death
Pt may admit to dangerous activities or preparing for death (e.g., giving away possessions, putting affairs in order, or new wills).

Is there a pt history or family history of psychologic disorders?
There is a genetic predisposition for depression.

Does the pt have a history of medical problems or drug abuse?
The symptoms cannot be caused by a medical or substance abuse problem.

Review current or past medications or supplements

 Check vital signs
Perform physical exam if symptoms suggest an organic cause
Perform mental status exam
General appearance and behavior: Check grooming, hygiene, attitude, psychomotor assessment, and eye contact.
Affect: Blunted, flat, or labile
Mood: Check for depressed mood.
Thought process: Assess speech and thoughts.
Thought content: Ask about suicide, hallucinations, delusions, and depersonalization.
Cognitive evaluation: Assess level of consciousness, orientation, attention and concentration, memory, basic knowledge, calculations, abstraction, insight, and judgment.

Consider the following labs:
CBC if signs of infection
Chemistry panel
RUDS if drug abuse
RPR to rule out syphilis if suspected
Serum alcohol level
TSH if suspect thyroid disease

Depression diagnosis has to meet the Diagnostic and Statistical Manual of Mental Disorder (DSM-IV) criteria:

Pt has to have either a depressed mood or loss of interest or pleasure.

Pt has to have a minimum of five of the following symptoms daily for a 2-week period, which also affect daily functioning:

- Depressed mood
- Hypersomnia or insomnia
- Loss of energy or fatigue
- Suicide ideation, plan, or attempt
- Excessive or inappropriate guilt or feelings of worthlessness
- Weight change without dieting
- Psychomotor retardation or agitation
- Inattention or inability to concentrate
- Less pleasure or interest in activities

The symptoms cannot be caused by a general medical condition, substance-induced mood disorder, or normal grieving as a result of the death of a loved one.

The symptoms cannot be caused by a psychotic disorder.

 Implement general measures

Allow pt to voice problems.

Be an attentive listener and remain as calm as possible.

Allow pt to be involved as much as possible in the care plan.

If suicidal:

- Discuss how much pain suicide would cause to loved ones.
- Pt has to be admitted with a psychiatric hold (usually 72 hours).

Start psychotherapy

Cognitive behavior therapy alone or in combination with medications

Start pharmacotherapy

SSRIs:
- Citalopram (Celexa)
- Sertraline (Zoloft)
- Paroxetine (Paxil)
- Fluoxetine (Prozac)
- Escitalopram (Lexapro)

Tricyclic antidepressants:
- Desipramine (Norpramin)
- Imipramine (Tofranil)
- Doxepin (Sinequan)
- Amitriptyline (Elavil)
- Nortriptyline (Aventyl, Pamelor)

Other classes:
- Bupropion (Wellbutrin)
- Nefazodone (Serzone)
- Trazodone (Desyrel)
- Tranylcypromine (Parnate)
- Mirtazapine (Remeron)
- Phenelzine (Nardil)
- Venlafaxine (Effexor)

Trial of electroconvulsive therapy if severe

Safe and very effective

Indicated in pts who are nonresponsive to medications, therapy, or at high risk for suicide

Educate pt and family about depression
Provide support groups that can be beneficial
Referral may be indicated in pts with comorbidities or complicated cases

S **Does the pt complain of sexual, physical, emotional, or verbal abuse?**
Take a complete and descriptive history of events and persons involved.

Provide an opportunity for the pt to give history alone.

Even if pt is married, there can still be sexual coercion or rape.
See Child Abuse (p. 184) and Elder Abuse (p. 192) for specifics on these types of abuse.

Is the history inconsistent with injuries?
Injury sustained may not be age appropriate or correlate with physical exam.
Suspicion should arise if pt delayed seeking medical care.

Did anyone witness the violence?
Document names of any witnesses or persons involved.

Ask the pt if it is safe to go home or if there are guns or weapons in the home
It is extremely important that you send the pt home to a safe place.

Ask about pt's past medical history or review chart
Pt may have a history of injuries over time that may be suspicious for abuse.
Review past medical history and medications.
Pt may have a medical condition that mimics abuse (see Child Abuse p. 184).

Assess risk factors that may indicate domestic violence
Risk factors may include pregnancy, relationship difficulty, financial problems, and/or
   recent divorce or separation.
See Child Abuse (p. 184) and Elder Abuse (p. 192) for specific risk factors in these
   groups.
Cultural, behavioral, psychiatric, or interpersonal factors may increase risk.

O **Check vital signs**
Perform physical exam
General:
   • Document any abnormalities.
   • Look for evidence of neglect.
HEENT:
   • Carefully examine the scalp.
   • Examine the eyes for retinal hemorrhages.
   • Check mouth for loose teeth or trauma.
   • Examine tympanic membranes for perforations.
Chest: Look for abnormal respirations.
Heart: Perform a complete heart exam.
Abdomen: Examine the groin area for abuse.
Genital: Refer to emergency room if suspected rape for rape kit collection; otherwise a
   full exam should be performed.
Extremities: Check pulses in upper and lower extremities.
Musculoskeletal:
   • Assess all joints for range of motion.
   • Refer to specific joint topic for a complete exam of joint in question.
   • Palpate for bony tenderness.
Neurologic: Perform complete exam, especially if head trauma is suspected.

Skin:
- Look for any lesions, such as bruises, in areas not normally seen:
  - Buttocks   - Ears   - Frenulum
  - Neck   - Thighs   - Torso
- Examine for burns that appear circumferential from immersion.
- Check for bite marks.
- Any lesion with well-demarcated shapes (e.g., belt buckle, cigarette, fist)
- Inspect for hand marks from grabbing.
- Look for lesions with multiple healing stages.
- Palpate all body surfaces.
- Photograph each lesion.

Consider the following labs and studies:
CBC if signs or symptoms of anemia or infection
PT/PTT if bruising or bleeding disorder suspected
X-rays of specific sites in questions
Skeletal survey if the child is less than 2 years old
CT scan of the head if suspected neurologic injury
Bone scan can be obtained in occult fractures.
Test for sexually transmitted infection if pt was raped.

 Domestic Violence

 Treat pt's injuries appropriately
Inform parents, caregiver, pt, or abuser about concern of abuse and steps required by law that must be taken to protect the pt
Notify police in all cases where abuse is suspected.
Notify Child Protective Services in all cases where children are involved.
Documentation is crucial and should be done carefully.

Place pt
Depending on findings, a medical decision needs to be made whether to hospitalize the pt, place in protective custody, or send home.
Pt and children can be placed in an emergency shelter that can also provide counseling.

Start intervention and support
Family, marriage, or couples counseling
The National Domestic Violence hotline can be helpful (1-800-799-SAFE)

S **Does the pt admit to drug use or have symptoms of drug use?**
Symptoms depend on the drug of choice.
See Alcoholism (p. 178) for specifics.
Dissociative drugs can cause hallucinations, rigidity, agitation, delusions, excitement, or fever.
Opiates usually cause euphoria, coma, hypotension, and respiratory depression.
Psychedelics can cause complaints of waking dreams, delusions, or hallucinations.
Stimulants may cause anxiety, diaphoresis, paranoia, hallucinations, hyperthermia, increased energy, decreased appetite, and cardiac symptoms.
Sedatives can present with respiratory depression, delirium, coma, or euphoria.

Are there symptoms of withdrawal?
Symptoms can include fatigue, hallucinations, hypotension, insomnia, seizures, cardiac symptoms, or nausea and vomiting.

Any psychological symptoms of depression, anxiety, psychosis, or manic states?
All drugs have the ability to cause psychological symptoms or exacerbate existing illnesses.
Pts with depression or anxiety may be self-treating with drugs.

Has drug use caused problems with the law, social life, work, or relationships?
Absenteeism, tardiness, frequent job changes, or decreased work productivity may be secondary to drug use.
Substance abuse is involved in more than half of motor vehicle deaths and domestic violence cases.
Sexual dysfunction, such as erectile dysfunction, may be related to drug abuse.

Does the pt have a medical problem caused by drug use?
A myriad of medical conditions can be associated with drug dependency.
Abusing drugs during pregnancy can be deleterious to the baby and mother.

Does the pt have a family history of alcohol or drug addiction?
There appears to be a genetic disposition for addiction.

O **Check vital signs**
Check for tachycardia, fever, or labile blood pressures, which may suggest withdrawal.

Perform physical exam
General:
- Check for gross defects, such as tremor or speech impediments.
- Observe for abnormal behavior.

HEENT:
- Check eyes for nystagmus, dilated, or constricted pupils.
- Observe for alcohol odor on breath.

Chest: Perform complete exam.
Heart: Check for tachycardia or displaced point of maximum impulse, which may indicate an enlarged heart.
Abdomen:
- Check for abdominal pain.
- Examine for an enlarged liver, ascites, or masses.

Skin:
- Look for spider angioma, caput medusae, and palmer erythema.
- Inspect for needle tracks or tattoos that cover tracks.

Consider the following labs and studies:
Serum alcohol level
RUDS if suspect other drugs

A **Drug Abuse**
Categories:

- Anabolic steroids	- Cannabinoids
- Dissociatives	- Opioids
- Psychedelics	- Sedative-hypnotics
- Stimulants	

P **Advise pt of your concerns**
Be nonjudgmental, empathetic, and nonconfrontational.
Depending on readiness of the pt, advise to cut down or stop all together.
Allow pt to be involved in planning and to set feasible goals.
Have close follow-up and congratulate pt if following treatment plan.

Refer to support groups such as:
Alcoholic Anonymous
Narcotics Anonymous
National Drug and Alcohol Treatment Referral Routing Service phone number:
- 1-800-662-HELP
Substance Abuse Facility Treatment Locator website:
- http://findtreatment.samhsa.gov

Refer to psychologist or psychiatrist if coexisting mental disorders are involved
Admit for detoxification to an inpatient or outpatient setting if necessary
Treat if signs of overdose
Anticholinergic drugs
- Treat overdose with physostigmine (Antilirium).
Cannabinoids
- Treatment is observation.
Dissociative
- Treat with haloperidol (Haldol) or risperidone (Risperdal).
Opiates
- Treat with tapering dose of methadone or clonidine.
- Naltrexone (Trexan) can be used to prevent pt from getting a high.
- Naloxone (Narcan) can be used to treat overdose.
Psychedelics
- Treatment is observation and possible psychiatric evaluation.
- Benzodiazepines and SSRIs can be used.
Sedative-hypnotics
- Phenobarbital and benzodiazepines can be used.
Stimulants
- Bromocriptine (Parlodel) and desipramine can be used in withdrawal.

S **Does the pt complain of abuse?**

Elderly pt may be subject to neglect, financial exploitation, violation of rights, or physical and/or psychologic abuse.

Review pt's financial situation.

Take a complete and descriptive history of events and persons involved.

Include a detailed description of the home or nursing home environment.

If possible, take separate histories from the caregiver and the pt.

Include in the histories all persons who care for the pt.

Obtain a history of the quality and nature of the relationship with the caregiver and whether the caregiver gives good care.

Is the history inconsistent with injuries?

Injury sustained may not be age appropriate or correlate with history or physical exam.

Suspicion should arise if caregiver delayed seeking medical care for the pt.

Caregiver may admit to inflicting injury on the pt.

Ask about pt's past medical history or review chart

The pt may have a history of injuries over time that is suspicious.

Review past medical history and medications.

Does the pt have a medical condition that may mimic elder abuse?

Refer to Child Abuse (p. 184) for list

Are there risk factors of elder abuse?

Risk factors include cognitive impairment, complicated medical conditions, unwanted or abandoned elder, or caregiver burnout.

Lack of adequate resources or education to take care of the pt

Caregivers under tremendous stress

Abuse of drugs or alcohol by the pt or caregiver

O **Check vital signs**
Perform physical exam

General:
- Document any abnormalities.
- Check for evidence of neglect, poor hygiene, or dehydration.

HEENT:
- Carefully examine the scalp.
- Check mouth for loose teeth or trauma.
- Examine tympanic membranes for perforations.

Chest: Look for abnormal respirations.

Heart: Perform a complete heart exam.

Abdomen: Examine the abdomen and genital area for abuse.

Extremities: Check pulses in upper and lower extremities.

Musculoskeletal:
- Assess joints for range of motion.
- Refer to specific joint topic for a complete exam of joint in question.
- Palpate for bony tenderness.

Neurologic: Full exam should be performed, especially in suspected head trauma.

Skin:
- Look for any lesions, such as bruises, in areas not normally seen:
  - Buttocks   - Ears   - Frenulum
  - Neck   - Thighs   - Torso
- Check for decubitus ulcers.
- Examine for burns that appear circumferential from immersion.
- Check for bite marks.
- Any lesion with well-demarcated shapes (e.g., belt buckle, cigarette, fist)
- Inspect for hand marks from grabbing.
- Look for lesions with multiple healing stages.
- Palpate all body surfaces.
- Photograph each lesion.

Consider the following labs and studies:
CBC if signs or symptoms of anemia or infection
PT/PTT if bruising or bleeding disorder is suspected
X-rays of specific sites in questions
CT scan of the head if suspected neurologic injury
Bone scan can be obtained in occult fractures

A   Elder Abuse

P   Treat pt's injuries appropriately
Inform caregiver, pt, or abuser about concern of abuse and steps required by law that must be taken to protect the pt
Notify Social Services and police in all cases where abuse is suspected.
Documentation is crucial and should be done carefully.
Competency of the pt should be determined.

Place pt
Depending on findings, a medical decision needs to be made whether to hospitalize the pt, place in protective custody, or send home with the caregiver.

Refer to senior advocacy groups
The National Domestic Violence hotline can be helpful (1-800-799-SAFE).

Index